Healthcare Access - New Threats, New Approaches

Edited by Ayşe Emel Önal

Published in London, United Kingdom

Healthcare Access - New Threats, New Approaches
http://dx.doi.org/10.5772/intechopen.104163
Edited by Ayşe Emel Önal

Contributors
Michael Mncedisi Willie, Thulisile Noutchang, Maninie Molatseli, Sipho Kabane, Ahmad Yahyq Alqassim, Maged El-Setouhy, Mxolisi Welcome Ngwenya, Gsakani Olivia Sumbane, Aaron Briggs, Malik Olatunde Oduoye, Aymar Akilimali, Umulkhairah Arama, Mohammed Fathelrahman Adam, Uwezo Biamba Chrispin, Bonk Muhoza Gasambi, Chakib Boukhalfa, Vivien O. Abah, Luis Augusto Moya-Barquín, Diana Leticia Coronel-Martínez, Robert Conrad Sierra Morales, Swapnil Morande, Kanwal Gul, Veena Tewari, Hilda Kawaya

First published in London, United Kingdom, 2023 by IntechOpen
IntechOpen is the global imprint of INTECHOPEN LIMITED, registered in England and Wales, registration number: 11086078, 5 Princes Gate Court, London, SW7 2QJ, United Kingdom

British Library Cataloguing-in-Publication Data
A catalogue record for this book is available from the British Library

Additional hard and PDF copies can be obtained from orders@intechopen.com

Healthcare Access - New Threats, New Approaches
Edited by Ayşe Emel Önal
p. cm.
Print ISBN 978-1-83768-161-7
Online ISBN 978-1-83768-162-4
eBook (PDF) ISBN 978-1-83768-163-1

For EU product safety concerns:
IN TECH d.o.o., Prolaz Marije Krucifikse Kozulić 3, 51000 Rijeka, Croatia,
info@intechopen.com or visit our website at intechopen.com.

Meet the editor

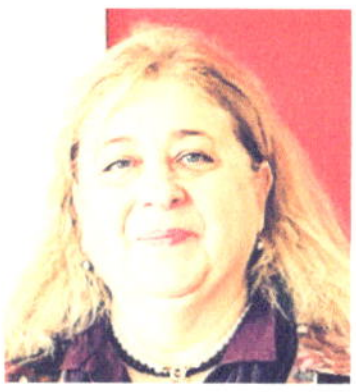

Ayşe Emel Önal graduated from the Istanbul Faculty of Medicine, Istanbul University, in 1995. In 1996, she became a public health specialist at the same university, followed by positions as a professor in 2011, head of the Department of Environmental Health in 2013, and head of the Department of Public Health in 2016. Her main research areas are communicable diseases, chronic non-communicable diseases, epidemiology, adolescent and youth health, gerontology, and environmental health. Dr. Önal has nearly 300 national and international

Contents

Preface

Access to health care is the ability to receive health services for the prevention, early detection, appropriate treatment, and tertiary prevention and care of diseases, disorders, and other conditions that affect health. For health care to be accessible, it must be affordable and able to protect and improve health. Today, it may not be possible to access health services in many parts of the world and in different settlements even within the same country. While this is common enough in Third World countries, it can also occur in developing and highly developed countries in certain circumstances such as disasters.

Governments, institutions, and health professionals are responsible for providing adequate health care. Access to health services becomes difficult in the face of economic problems, conflicts, global climate change, internal and external migrations, beliefs, and so on. This book discusses both barriers to and opportunities for accessing health services. If the barriers are poverty, illiteracy, and false beliefs, the opportunities may be organization, communication, stratification of health care, and categorization and training of health workers to reach homes at one end and to practice personalized medicine at the other. This book includes ten chapters over four sections.

Section I, "Environment – Health Relationship and Access to Health Services", includes two chapters: Chapter 1: "Impact of Poverty on Health" and Chapter 2: "Climate Change, Conflict, and Contagion: Emerging Threats to Global Public Health".

Section II, "Access to Health Services for Important Health Problems", includes four chapters that discuss common diseases that kill, disable, and cause the most workday loss: Chapter 3: "Funding of Oncology Benefits by Medical Schemes, South Africa: A Focus on Breast and Cervical Cancer", Chapter 4: "Healthcare Services for the Physically Challenged Persons in Africa: Challenges and Way Forward", Chapter 5: "The Urgency of Access to Men-Centered Mental Healthcare Services to Address Men's Sensitive Issues in the Communities of South Africa" and Chapter 6: "The 4H and 4T Pediatric Early Acute Support in the Deteriorating Child: Competent Staff Instead Experts Facing the New Threats, and New Approaches Can Reduce Mortality – Experience in Guatemala".

Section III, "Barriers and Opportunities to Access to Health Care and Universal Health Coverage", includes three chapters: Chapter 7: "The Road to Universal Coverage by the End of 2022, the Moroccan Challenge", Chapter 8: "Poor Health Care Access in Nigeria: A Function of Fundamental Misconceptions and Misconstruction of the Health System" and Chapter 9: "Home Visitation by Community Health Workers".

Section IV, "Artificial Intelligence and Telemedicine in Health Care", includes the final chapter: Chapter 10: "Reinforcing Positive Cognitive States with Machine Learning: An Experimental Modeling for Preventive Healthcare".

Global and regional income inequality, wars caused by unshared energy, air, and water, and soil pollution caused by fossil fuels, global climate change, natural disasters, and other factors increase acute and chronic health problems in the world and make it difficult to access health services. Economic deprivations prevent access to water, sanitation, and hygiene, and increase food insecurity and deaths from infections. Economic deprivation also weakens health infrastructure. Therefore, it becomes difficult both to receive preventive health services and appropriate treatment. This book opens new horizons in accessing health services.

I would like to thank our esteemed authors for their excellent contributions and the staff at IntechOpen for selecting me as editor and for their invaluable assistance throughout the publication process.

Ayşe Emel Önal
Professor, MD,
Public Health Specialist,
Istanbul University,
Istanbul Medical Faculty,
Istanbul, Türkiye

Section 1

Environment – Health Relationship and Access to Health Services

Chapter 1

Impact of Poverty on Health

Ahmad Alqassim and Maged El-Setouhy

Abstract

Poverty is not merely the absence of money but the absence of resources to get the necessities of life. Poverty and health are always in a reciprocal relationship. This relation came to light in 1948 when the WHO defined health as complete physical, mental and social well-being. In 1987, the Alma Ata Declaration opened the discussion on health inequity. This opened the door for thousands of projects, proposals, and publications on this relation. Although the relationship between poverty and infectious diseases was clear, there was inequity in funding. The Global Fund invests US$ 4 billion annually for AIDS, tuberculosis, and Malaria, while other diseases lack funds. That is why they were considered neglected tropical diseases. However, the relationship between health and poverty is not limited to infectious diseases but includes noninfectious problems like malnutrition and injuries. In this chapter, we will assess the association between poverty as a predictor and health as an outcome.

Keywords: poverty, infectious diseases, malnutrition, developing countries, public health

1. Introduction

There are several definitions of poverty as a concept based on the context of the topic in which it is placed. During the World Summit on Social Development in Copenhagen in 1995, 117 countries adopted two concepts for poverty absolute and overall [1]. An ambitious global plan was proposed to eliminate absolute poverty and reduce overall poverty. Absolute poverty was defined as "a condition characterized by severe deprivation of basic human needs, including food, safe drinking water, sanitation facilities, health, shelter, education, and information. It depends not only on income but also on access to services." On the other hand, overall poverty is a "lack of income and productive resources to ensure sustainable livelihoods; hunger and malnutrition; ill health; limited or lack of access to education and other basic services; increased morbidity and mortality from illness; homelessness and inadequate housing; unsafe environments and social discrimination and exclusion. It is also characterized by a lack of participation in decision-making and civil, social, and cultural life. It occurs in all countries: as mass poverty in many developing countries, pockets of poverty amid wealth in developed countries, loss of livelihoods as a result of economic recession, sudden poverty as a result of disaster or conflict, the poverty of low-wage workers, and the utter lack of people who fall outside family support systems, social institutions and safety nets.".

Every country has its concept of poverty. However, the world bank defined poverty as "Poverty is a pronounced deprivation in well-being." [2].

Traditional poverty is a lack of essential resources for basic needs such as hygienic food, water, clothing, and shelter. However, access to healthcare, education, and transportation might also be included as indicators of poverty in the modern world. In general, Poverty is a state in which a community or person lacks the Necessary needs for minimal standard of living in that place.

2. Global poverty lines

Each country has its own definition of poverty. The poverty line is substantially lower in poorer countries than in richer ones [3]. This means that if we were to only depend on national poverty criteria for a global measure of poverty, the outcome would be a measuring framework in which a person's place of residence would decide whether or not they were poor. Setting global poverty lines based on national definitions and applying them globally is one solution to this issue. The global Poverty Line was determined in this manner by the United Nations. The global poverty line must be frequently adjusted to account for changes in worldwide price disparities. The new global poverty line was updated to $2.15 starting in the fall of 2022 [4]. Therefore, it is considered extreme poverty for someone to make less than $2.15 daily.

3. Poverty facts

More than 689 million people rely on less than $1.9 per day, while 250 million are under the global poverty line [5]. Two-thirds of the world's poor people are children and young, while women predominate in most areas [6]. Sub-Saharan Africa sees an increase in the concentration of extreme poverty, and about A little over 40% of the local population makes less than $1.90 each day [7]. Between 2015 and 2018, the Middle East and North Africa experienced a nearly doubling of the extreme poverty rate, from 3.8 to 7.2%, primarily due to the political conflicts in the area [8]. Between 2015 and 2018, the Middle East and North Africa experienced a nearly doubling of the extreme poverty rate, from 3.8 to 7.2%, primarily due to the political conflicts in the area [9]. Around 67% of the world's poor people are predicted to live in unstable regions by 2030 [9]. In extreme poverty, 70% of adults over 15 either have no formal or minimal education. Around 1.3 billion people reside in 107 developing nations and experience poverty [10].

4. Poverty and health

Globally, poverty and poor health are deeply associated [11]. Disparities in politics, society, and the economy are the underlying causes of poor health among millions worldwide. Poverty is both a cause and a consequence of poor health [12]. Infectious and neglected tropical diseases affect millions of the world's poorest and most vulnerable individuals annually [13]. Poverty is a crucial contributor to poor health and a barrier to receiving necessary medical care [14]. Financial restrictions prevent poor people from acquiring the necessities for optimal health, such as enough quantity of high-quality food and medical care. However, the relationship is also linked to other aspects of poverty, such as a lack of knowledge about the best ways to promote health or a lack of a voice to ensure that social services are effective for them. Because they lack the knowledge, resources, or access to healthcare that would enable them to prevent and treat disease, marginalized groups and vulnerable individuals frequently suffer the most. Indigenous communities and other marginalized groups may have severe health repercussions due to reduced healthcare use due to cultural and social barriers, which maintain their extreme poverty levels [15]. Robust health systems protect populations from the potentially disastrous effects of out-of-pocket healthcare costs and enhance the entire population's health status, especially the poor, who are more likely to experience poor health and limited access to healthcare [16]. In general, the poor are disproportionately more likely to have bad health [17].

5. Ending poverty's current challenges

Globally, the number of people suffering from extreme poverty, poor people living on less than $1.90 a day, decreased from 36% in 1990 to only 10% in 2015 [12]. For nearly 25 years, the number of poor people living on less than $1.90 a day has been steadily declining [18]. Unfortunately, this gradual improvement was halted in 2020 by the effects of the COVID-19 pandemic [19]. The COVID-19 pandemic has swept back decades of progress in the fight against poverty. According to the World Bank, the COVID-19 pandemic pushed between 143 and 163 million people in 2021 into extreme poverty [20]. Some countries have been affected more than others. We find that countries in South Asia and Sub-Saharan Africa have suffered from new waves of high extreme poverty rates, more than previously reported [21]. These large numbers of these "new poor" will be in addition to the already 1.3 billion poor people living in extreme poverty and experiencing exacerbated life difficulties in light of the COVID-19 pandemic [22]. Poverty rates are alarmingly high, especially in developing countries that are the most vulnerable to economic risks since the onset of the COVID-19 pandemic [23]. These devastating effects on developing countries are not just due to health crises but also because of the pandemic's impact as a devastating social and economic crisis for the foreseeable future [24]. According to the United Nations Development Program, income losses are expected to exceed $220 billion in developing countries [12]. The world's population without access to social protection is expected to reach an estimated 5% of people [25]. All this will lead to the repercussions of these losses affecting education, human rights, basic food security, and global nutrition. There is a light at the end of the tunnel due to the beginning of the recovery phase from the pandemic starting in 2022 [26]. This might contribute to returning to the right track in achieving sustainable development goals in many countries where poverty rates have risen to record numbers [12]. These record numbers caused mistrust of these countries in the current global sustainable development plans. The need has become urgent and intense to start taking actual steps by developed countries to reduce poverty rates by opening economic cooperation and transferring sufficient expertise to improve the economic environment for these countries.

6. Diseases related to poverty

As described above, poverty and ill health are mutually related as each affects the other. Infectious diseases are mostly related to poverty, so we will only consider them in this chapter. Aiming to integrate health with the plans to eradicate poverty, the World Health Organization developed the International Poverty and Health network in 1997. This network of people and organizations from business, health, governmental and non-governmental organizations worked on developing policies to improve the health of the poor populations worldwide [27].

Three years later, with the support of the Group of eight (G8) (Group of eight, namely the United States, Canada, the United Kingdom, France, Germany, Japan, Italy, and Russia), the global fund was declared to cover three diseases that appear as unstopped in different countries. The Global Fund invests US$ 4 billion annually for AIDS, Tuberculosis, and Malaria, while many other diseases lack funds for eradication or elimination.

That is why they were called neglected tropical diseases, mainly prevalent in the tropical and subtropical regions of Africa, Asia, and the Americas. However, they included a group of infectious diseases that are highly prevalent in these developing countries. These three events and declarations defined the diseases concerning poverty. But unfortunately, the first three Malaria, Tuberculosis, and HIV/AIDS were lucky to get the global fund, while others were neglected as defined.

To make it easy, we divided poverty-related diseases into two main groups those covered by the Global Fund and those considered neglected tropical diseases.

6.1 Diseases covered by the global fund

Replace the entirety of this text with the main body of your chapter. The body is where the author explains experiments, presents and interprets data of one's research. Authors are free to decide how the main body will be structured. However, you are required to have at least one heading. Please ensure that either British or American English is used consistently in your chapter.

6.1.1 HIV/AIDS

After the death of the first known case of HIV/AIDS in Kinshasa (Belonging to Congo nowadays) in Africa in 1959, the disease spread to many other countries in the world as a global blood-born and sexually transmitted disease pandemic (**Figures 1** and **2**) (**Table 1**) [28]. The estimated number of globally infected people now is around 38 million [29]. The virus attacks the immune system with different manifestations of the disease ranging from the carrier state with no manifestations to severe immune-depression states and death. No standard curative treatment is known for the disease [30–33]. That is why the patients' early diagnosis, symptomatic treatment, and care help them to live longer. However, primary prevention is considered the cornerstone in preventing the spread of the disease [34–36].

This would describe the much higher prevalence of deaths from HIV/AIDS in developing countries compared to developed countries and even the higher deaths in the developed countries among poor people who have limited access to healthcare facilities [37–42]. This fact is evident in maps 1 and 2 quoted from the WHO website 2017, especially compared to the extreme poverty presented earlier (**Figure 3**), where Africa carries the primary disease burden and deaths from the disease [43].

That is why the global health sector strategies (GHSSs) focus on HIV, viral hepatitis, and sexually transmitted infections for 2022–2030. The GHSSs guide the health sector in implementing strategically focused responses to end AIDS,

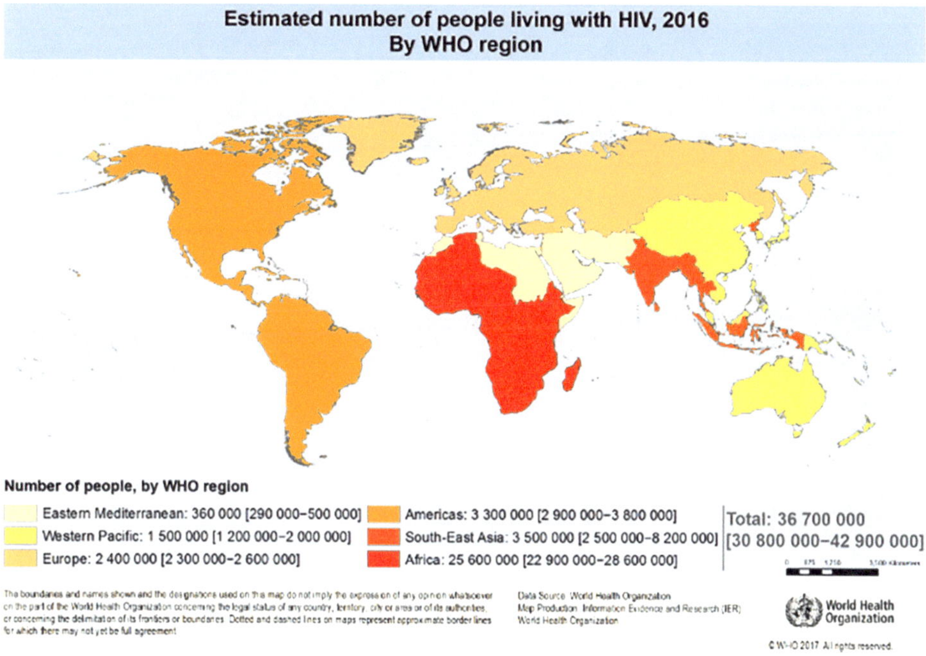

Figure 1.
The global estimated number of people living with HIV, 2016. Source: WHO/UNAIDS/UNICEF©.

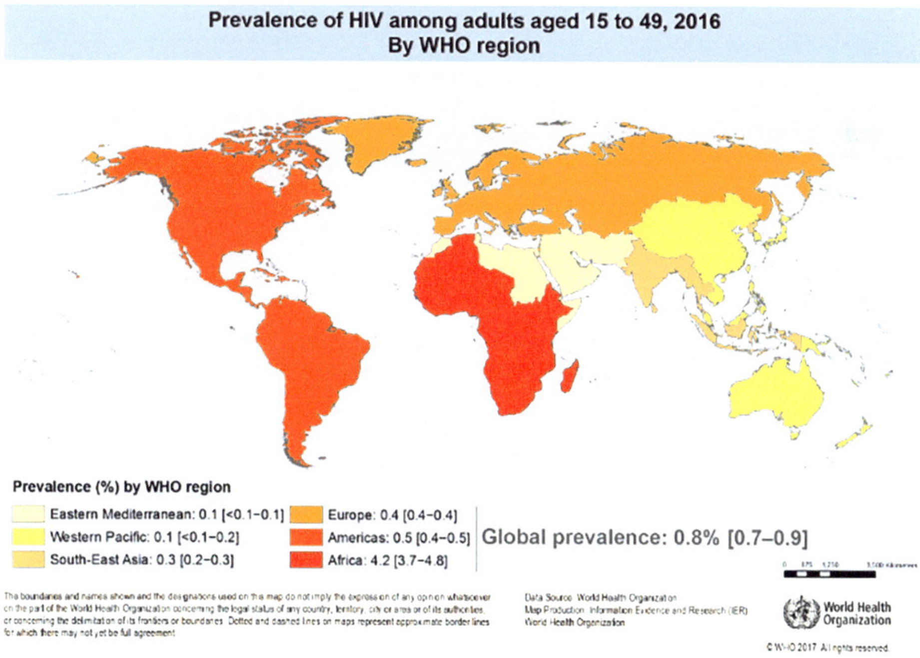

Figure 2.
The global prevalence of HIV among adults aged 15 to 49, 2016. Source: WHO/UNAIDS/UNICEF©.

Summary of the global HIV epidemic, 2021

	People living with HIV in 2021	People acquiring HIV in 2021	People dying from HIV-related causes in 2021
Total	38.4 million [33.9–43.8 million]	1.5 million [1.1–2.0 million]	650 000 [510 000–860 000]
Adults (15+ years)	36.7 million [32.3–41.9 million]	1.3 million [990 000–1.8 million]	560 000 [430 000–740 000]
Women (15+ years)	19.7 million [17.6–22.4 million]	640 000 [480 000–870 000]	240 000 [180 000–320 000]
Men (15+ years)	16.9 million [14.6–19.7 million]	680 000 [500 000–920 000]	320 000 [250 000–430 000]
Children (<15 years)	1.7 million [1.3–2.1 million]	160 000 [110 000–230 000]	98 000 [67 000–140 000]

Source: UNAIDS/WHO estimates

Updated: July 2022

World Health Organization

Table 1.
The global burden of the HIV epidemic, 2021. Source: WHO©.

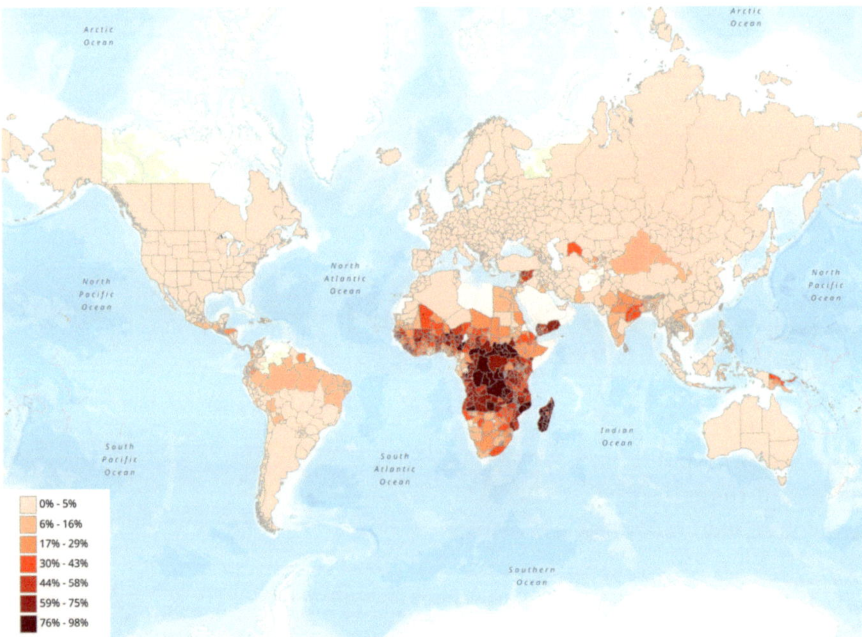

Figure 3.
Poverty proportion at $1.90 a day, 2018. Source: World Bank©, Poverty Global Practice, and Development Economics Division. Data are based on household survey data obtained from different government statistical agencies and the World Bank country departments.

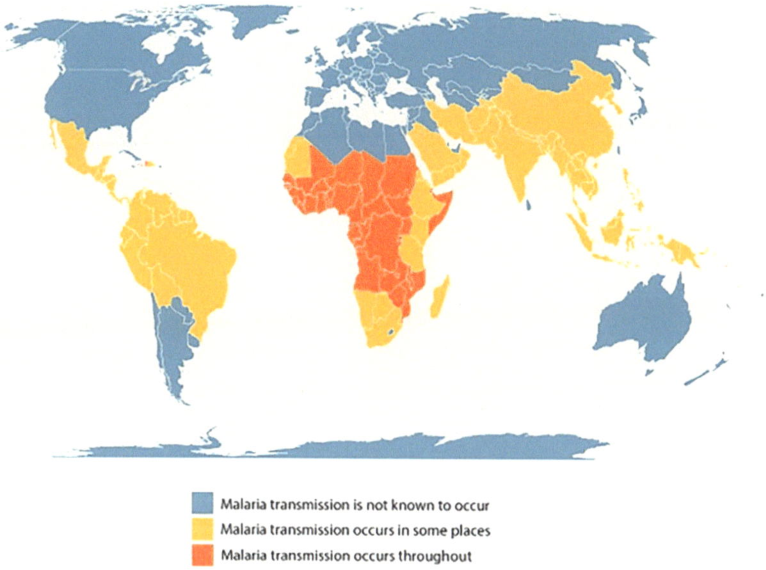

Figure 4.
The global endemic locations for malaria worldwide, 2020. Source: Global Health, Division of Parasitic Diseases and Malaria, CDC©.

viral hepatitis B and C, and sexually transmitted infections by 2030. This would be achieved through the synergistic work of different health sectors with the Primary Health Care (PHC) [44].

6.1.2 Malaria

Malaria is a vector-borne parasitic disease transmitted by anopheline mosquitos [45, 46]. The disease is caused mainly by four kinds of malaria parasites that can affect man. They are called Plasmodium (P) falciparum, P. vivax, P. oval, and P. malariae [47]. The estimated number of Malaria cases in 2020 was 241 million in 85 endemic countries. The global Malaria map (**Figure 4**) is nearly the same as the poverty map presented earlier. Malaria is mainly prevalent in poor countries [48]. Most Malaria cases (around 95%) are present in Africa [49]. Although most developed countries eliminated the disease, developing countries did not [50, 51].

The World Health Organization (WHO) launched the first Global Malaria Eradication Program (GMEP) in 1955 [52]. The program targeted The Americas, Europe, and Asia through spraying DDT and the use of chloroquine [53, 54]. However, most African countries were excluded due to logistical difficulties at that time (most of them were occupied by European countries) [55, 56]. However, in 1969, the WHO suspended this program after developing resistance to the treatment and the insecticides [57]. Malaria re-emerged in Europe in the 1990s, and the WHO launched the Roll Back Malaria program in 1998 using insecticides that impregnated bed nets and new cheap drugs [52, 58–60]. In 1987 Mosquirix vaccine was created against P. falciparum malaria and hepatitis B after great efforts and funds. The vaccine is now available in Europe for children aged 6 weeks to 17 months, but not yet for poor African children, although Africa carried all the burden of the vaccine's clinical trials [61–63]. Although malaria is eradicated in

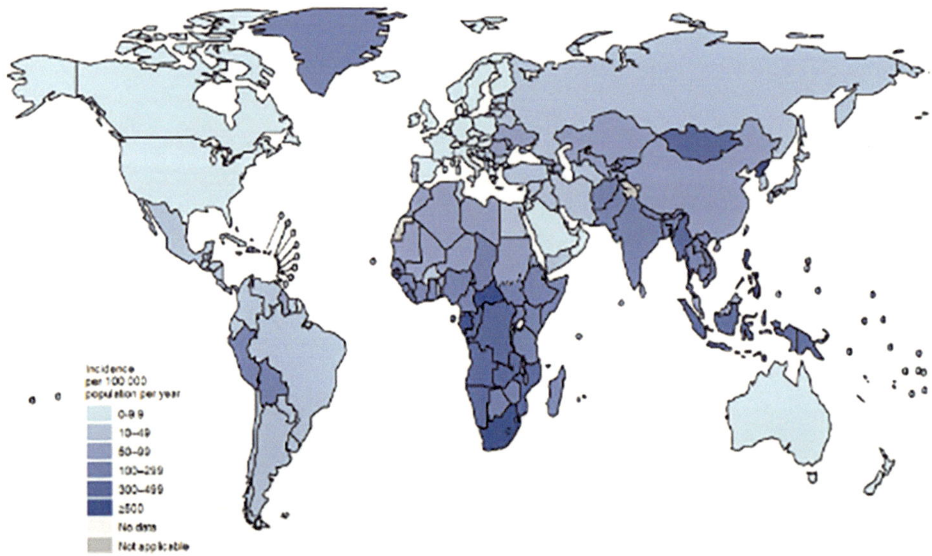

Figure 5.
The global estimated TB incidence rates, 2020. Source: Global Tuberculosis Report 2021, WHO©.

the United States and most of the European countries, it is still highly prevalent in the poor countries of Africa [52].

6.1.3 Tuberculosis

Tuberculosis (TB) is one of the oldest diseases caused by tubercle bacilli. It is a disease in poor people and countries. It is highly prevalent in developing countries, as shown in the map compared with the poverty map [64–67]. Despite all efforts to eradicate tuberculosis (TB), it remains a threat to global health (**Figure 5**). In the early 1920s, the BCG vaccine against tuberculosis was available. However, no universal global vaccination program has been adopted, and still, tuberculosis is responsible for millions of deaths [68]. Different lines of treatment were developed to eliminate the disease, as drug resistance developed for some medications used to treat the disease [69, 70]. However, Directly Observed Therapy (DOT) is still effective in many areas but in poor areas where direct observation of the therapy is impossible [71–73]. The concurrent infection with HIV in poor areas was a decisive factor hindering the disease treatment [74]. Poverty with overcrowding, inadequate housing, poor ventilation, and famines were all contributing factors to the disease's continued among poor populations.

6.2 Neglected tropical diseases related to poverty

Neglected tropical diseases (NTDs) are affecting more than 1 billion propel. They are mainly diseases of poor populations in the tropical and subtropical areas [75, 76]. They are a group of 20 diseases as mentioned down:

- Buruli ulcer
- Chagas disease

- Dengue and chikungunya
- Dracunculiasis
- Echinococcosis
- Foodborne trematodiases
- Human African trypanosomiasis
- Leishmaniasis
- Leprosy
- Lymphatic filariasis
- Rabies
- Mycetoma, chromoblastomycosis and other deep mycoses
- Onchocerciasis
- Scabies and other ectoparasitoses
- Schistosomiasis
- Soil-transmitted helminthiases
- Snakebite envenoming
- Taeniasis and cysticercosis
- Trachoma
- Yaws

The NTDs are mainly diseases in developing countries, as shown in the maps of some of the NTDs down if compared to the map of poverty shown earlier in the chapter (**Figure 6**) [77–84]. However, due to a lack of funding, the WHO published a 2021 booklet as a road to end the NTDs by 2030 by integrating their prevention and control (**Figure 7**) [76].

As described above and with comparing the maps of the diseases described it is obvious that fighting poverty should be considered in preventing these diseases (**Figure 8**). Whatever we would do to prevent these diseases, they will continue affecting poor people till poverty is controlled (**Figure 9**).

7. Conclusion

Poverty is the economic condition in which the individual lacks sufficient income to obtain the minimum levels of food, clothing, healthcare, education, and all the

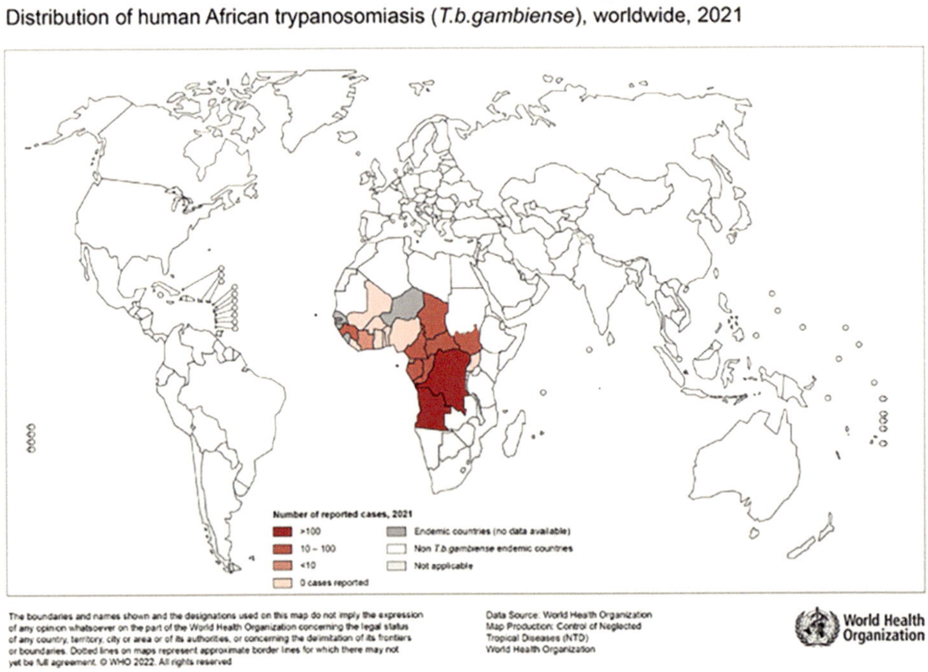

Figure 6.
The global distribution of human African trypanosomiasis, 2021. Source: WHO©.

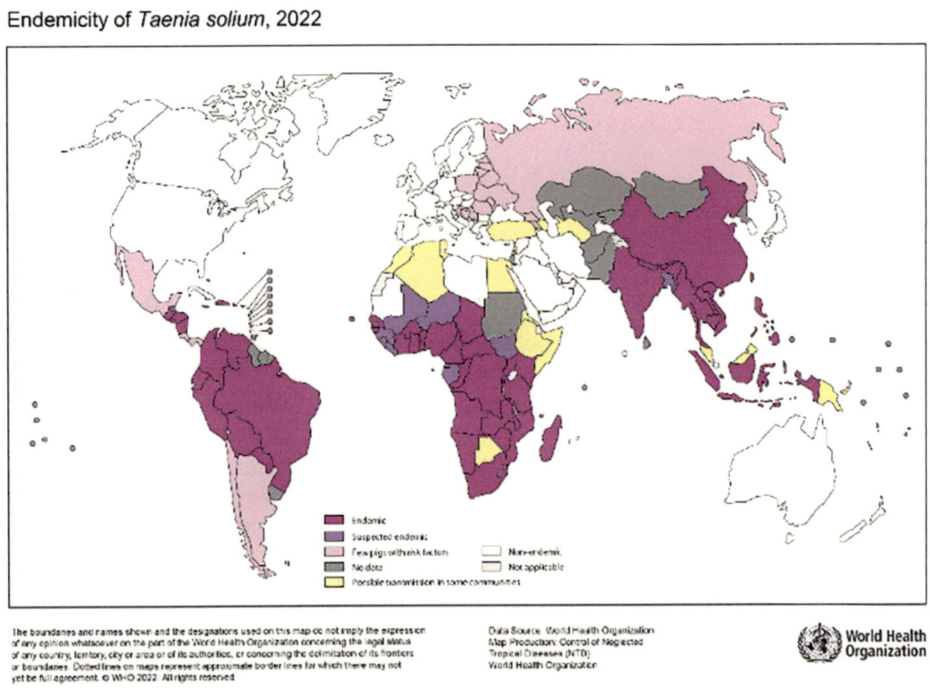

Figure 7.
The global endemic locations for Taenia solium, 2022. Source: WHO©.

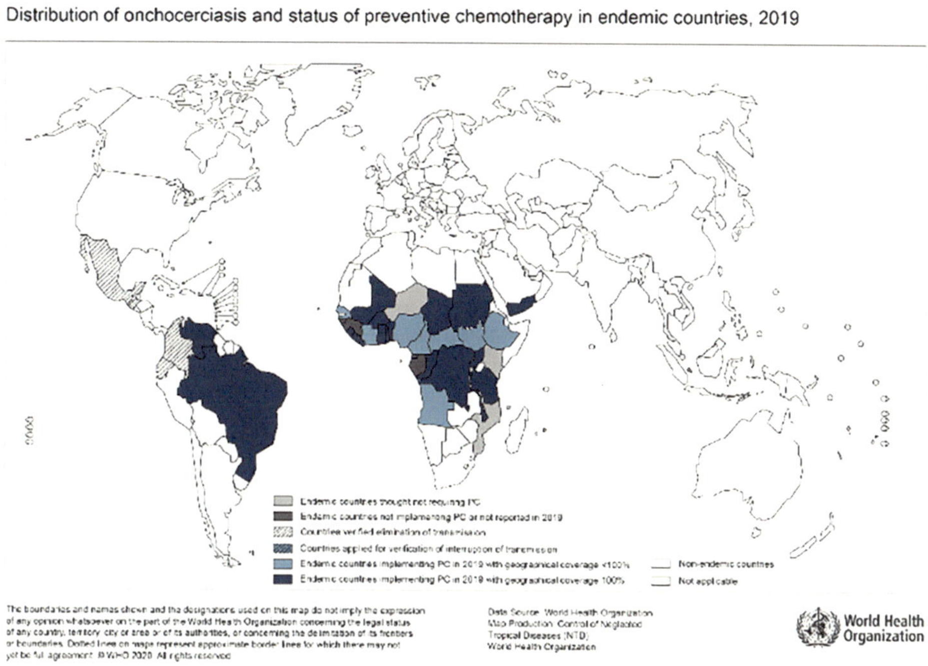

Figure 8.
The global endemic locations for onchocerciasis and the status of its preventive chemotherapy, 2019. Source: WHO©.

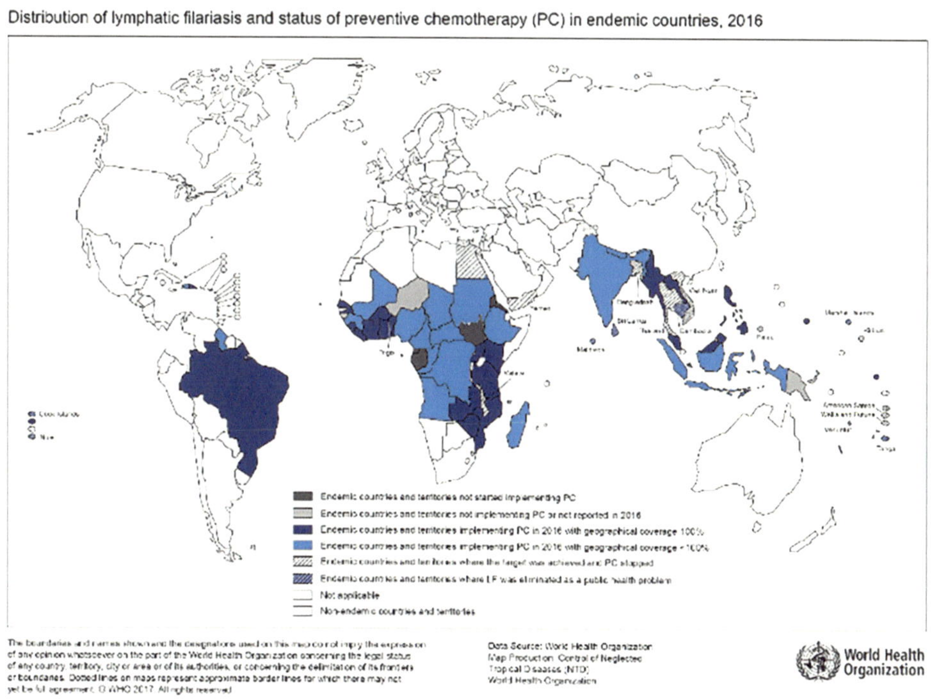

Figure 9.
The global endemic locations for lymphatic filariasis and the status of its preventive chemotherapy, 2016. Source: WHO©.

needs necessary to secure a decent standard of life. The phenomenon of poverty in all countries of the world is considered an intractable problem. However, in developing countries, the significant increase in poverty rates is the problem. In addition, the COVID-19 pandemic has dramatically affected the increase in poverty rates, especially in developing countries.

Poverty affects health significantly in several directions. Malnutrition is when the poor suffer from the lack of food, and it may not be healthy if available. They also suffer from malnutrition, which makes children starve to death. The inability to access healthcare, as the poor cannot afford the healthcare expenses or buy the medications they need, is a considerable obstacle. Poverty is associated with a higher risk of diseases, epidemics, and early deaths. The relationship between poverty with health remains a deep-rooted relationship, no matter how researchers differ in determining who affects the other. Therefore, developed countries must increase the rates of economic cooperation and support the development of developing countries.

Acknowledgements

We would like to extend our sincere thanks to international and local organizations such as the United Nations, World Bank, and CDC for making valuable data and information available to researchers and supporting developing countries' development process.

Conflict of interest

The authors declare no conflict of interest.

Author details

Ahmad Alqassim* and Maged El-Setouhy
Faculty of Medicine, Family and Community Medicine Department, Jazan University, Jazan, Saudi Arabia

*Address all correspondence to: ahmadalqassim1407@gmail.com

References

[1] United Nations. The Copenhagen Declaration and Programme of Action: World Summit for Social Development 6-12 March 1995. New York: United Nations Department of Publications; 1995

[2] World Bank. World Development Report 2000/2001: Attacking Poverty. Washington, DC: World Bank; 2000

[3] Jolliffe D, Prydz EB. Estimating international poverty lines from comparable national thresholds. The Journal of Economic Inequality. 2016;**14**(2):185-198

[4] De F, Fu H, Sànchez-Pàramo C. An Adjustment to Global Poverty Lines. The World Bank Group; 2022. Available from: https://blogs.worldbank.org/voices/adjustment-global-poverty-lines

[5] Kagimu I. Sustainable rural poverty alleviation programs: A case study of Uganda [Doctoral thesis]. 2022;**1**(1):1-48

[6] Olinto P, Beegle K, Sobrado C, Uematsu H. The state of the poor: Where are the poor, where is extreme poverty harder to end, and what is the current profile of the world's poor. Economic premise. 2013;**125**(2):1-8

[7] Schoch M, Lakner C. The Number of Poor People Continues to Rise in Sub-Saharan Africa, Despite a Slow Decline in the Poverty Rate. The World Bank Group; 2020. Available from: https://blogs.worldbank.org/opendata/number-poor-people-continues-rise-sub-saharan-africa-despite-slow-decline-poverty-rate

[8] Castaneda Aguilar RA, Cojocaru A, Howton ELA, Lakner C, Nguyen MC, Schoch M, et al. Poverty and Shared Prosperity 2020: Reversals of Fortune. The World Bank Group; 2020. Available from: https://www.worldbank.org/en/publication/poverty-and-shared-prosperity-2020

[9] World Bank. Monvitoring Global Poverty. Poverty and Shared Prosperity 2020: Reversals of Fortune: The World Bank Group; 2020. p. 27-80. Available from: https://elibrary.worldbank.org/doi/abs/10.1596/978-1-4648-1602-4_ch1

[10] Alkire S, Dirksen J, Nogales R, Oldiges C. Multidimensional poverty and COVID-19 risk factors: A rapid overview of interlinked deprivations across 5.8 billion people. 2020

[11] Chokshi DA. Income, poverty, and health inequality. Journal of the American Medical Association. 2018;**319**(13):1312-1313

[12] UN. Sustainable Development Goals. Goal 1: End poverty in all its forms everywhere. United Nations: United Nations Publications; 2022. Available from: https://www.un.org/sustainabledevelopment/poverty/

[13] Feasey N, Wansbrough-Jones M, Mabey DC, Solomon AW. Neglected tropical diseases. British Medical Bulletin. 2010;**93**(1):179-200

[14] WHO. Poverty and Health. The World Bank Group; 2003. Available from: https://www.worldbank.org/en/topic/health/brief/poverty-health

[15] United Nations. Mandated Areas: Health. United Nations: United Nations Publications; 2022. Available from: https://www.un.org/development/desa/indigenouspeoples/mandated-areas1/health.html

[16] Sirag A, Mohamed NN. Out-of-pocket health expenditure and poverty: Evidence from a dynamic panel

threshold analysis. Healthcare (Basel). 2021;**9**(5):1-20

[17] Gupta RP, de Wit ML, McKeown D. The impact of poverty on the current and future health status of children. Paediatrics & Child Health. 2007;**12**(8):667-672

[18] World Bank. Decline of Global Extreme Poverty Continues but Has Slowed: World Bank [press release]. Washington, D.C.: The World Bank Group; 2018

[19] Pereira M, Oliveira AM. Poverty and food insecurity may increase as the threat of COVID-19 spreads. Public health nutrition. 2020;**23**(17):3236-3240

[20] Lanker C, Yonzan N, Mahler G, Aguilar RAC, Wu H. Updated estimates of the impact of COVID-19 on global poverty: Looking back at 2020 and the outlook for 2021. 2021

[21] Aguilar RAC, Diaz-Bonilla C, Fujs T, Lakner C, Mahler DG, Nguyen MC, et al. September 2022 global poverty update from the World Bank: 2017 PPPs and new data for India. The World Bank Group; 2022. Available from: https://blogs.worldbank.org/opendata/september-2022-global-poverty-update-world-bank-2017-ppps-and-new-data-india

[22] United Nations. International Day for the Eradication of Poverty 2021. United Nations; 2021. Available from: https://www.un.org/development/desa/socialperspectiveondevelopment/international-day-for-the-eradication-of-poverty-homepage/2021-2.html

[23] Sánchez-Páramo C, Hill R, Mahler DG, Narayan A, Yonzan N. COVID-19 Leaves a Legacy of Rising Poverty and Widening Inequality. The World Bank Groups; 2021. Available from: https://blogs.worldbank.org/developmenttalk/covid-19-leaves-legacy-rising-poverty-and-widening-inequality

[24] OECD. The impact of the coronavirus (COVID-19) crisis on development finance. OECD Policy Responses to Coronavirus (COVID-19). 2020

[25] Spasova S, Bouget D, Ghailani D, Vanhercke B. Access to social protection for people working on non-standard contracts and as self-employed in Europe. A study of national policies Brussels: European Commission. 2017

[26] del Rio C, Malani PN. COVID-19 in 2022—The beginning of the end or the end of the beginning? Journal of the American Medical Association. 2022;**327**(24):2389-2390

[27] Haines A, Heath I, Smith R. Joining together to combat poverty. Everybody welcome and needed. BMJ. 2000;**320**(7226):1-2

[28] de Sousa JD, Muller V, Lemey P, Vandamme AM. High GUD incidence in the early 20 century created a particularly permissive time window for the origin and initial spread of epidemic HIV strains. PLoS One. 2010;**5**(4):e9936

[29] WHO. The Global Health Observatory: WHO; 2022 [updated July 2022; cited 2022 Sept. 10]. HIV data]. Available from: https://www.who.int/data/gho/data/themes/hiv-aids#:~:text=Globally%2C%2038.4%20million%20%5B33.9%E2%80%93,considerably%20between%20countries%20and%20regions.

[30] Islam RK, Donnelly E, Islam KN. Circulating hydrogen sulfide (H_2S) and nitric oxide (NO) levels are significantly reduced in HIV patients concomitant with increased oxidative stress biomarkers. Journal of Clinical Medicine. 2021;**10**(19):1-13

[31] Ning S, Zeng C, Zeng C, Zhao Y. The TAR binding dynamics and its implication in Tat degradation

mechanism. Biophysical Journal. 2021;**120**(23):5158-5168

[32] Vanangamudi M, Nair PC, Engels SEM, Palaniappan S, Namasivayam V. Structural insights to human immunodeficiency virus (HIV-1) targets and their inhibition. Advances in Experimental Medicine and Biology. 2021;**1322**:63-95

[33] Weldemariam SA, Dagnew Z, Tafere Y, Bereka TM, Bitewa YB. Time to death among HIV-infected under-five children after initiation of anti-retroviral therapy and its predictors in Oromiya liyu zone, Amhara region, Ethiopia: A retrospective cohort study. BMC Pediatrics. 2022;**22**(1):5

[34] Mambanga P, Sirwali RN, Tshitangano T. Factors contributing to men's reluctance to seek HIV counselling and testing at primary health care facilities in vhembe district of South Africa. African Journal of Primary Health Care & Family Medicine. 2016;**8**(2):e1-e7

[35] Rietmeijer CA. Improving care for sexually transmitted infections. Journal of the International AIDS Society. 2019;**22**(Suppl 6):e25349

[36] Tshweneagae GT, Oss VM, Mgutshini T. Disclosure of HIV status to sexual partners by people living with HIV. Curationis. 2015;**38**(1)

[37] Attal BA, Al-Rowaishan KM, Akeel AA, AlAmmar FK. HIV stigma in the teaching hospitals in Sana'a, Yemen: A conflict and low-resource setting. BMC Public Health. 2021;**21**(1):1793

[38] Bousmah MA, Nishimwe ML, Kuaban C, Boyer S. Free access to antiretroviral treatment and protection against the risk of catastrophic health expenditure in people living with HIV: Evidence from Cameroon. BMC Health Services Research. 2021;**21**(1):313

[39] Gwako GN, Were F, Obimbo MM, Kinuthia J, Gachuno OW, Gichangi PB. Association between utilization and quality of antenatal care with stillbirths in four tertiary hospitals in a low-income urban setting. Acta Obstetricia et Gynecologica Scandinavica. 2021;**100**(4):676-683

[40] Onyango DO, van der Sande MAB, Musingila P, Kinywa E, Opollo V, Oyaro B, et al. High HIV prevalence among decedents received by two high-volume mortuaries in Kisumu, western Kenya, 2019. PLoS One. 2021;**16**(7):e0253516

[41] Pahwa S, Deeks S, Zou S, Tomitch N, Miller-Novak L, Caler E, et al. NIH Workshop on HIV-associated comorbidities, coinfections, and complications: Summary and recommendation for future research. Journal of Acquired Immune Deficiency Syndromes. 2021;**86**(1):11-18

[42] Yang X, Li X, Qiao S, Shen Z, Zhou Y. Socioeconomic disparity of immunologic outcome among people living with HIV in Guangxi, China. AIDS Care. 2021;**33**(3):347-351

[43] Parker E, Judge MA, Macete E, Nhampossa T, Dorward J, Langa DC, et al. HIV infection in Eastern and Southern Africa: Highest burden, largest challenges, greatest potential. Southern African Journal of HIV Medicine. 2021;**22**(1):1237

[44] World Health Organization. Global Health Sector Strategies on, Respectively, HIV, Viral Hepatitis and Sexually Transmitted Infections for the Period 2022-2030. World Health Organization; 2022. p. 134. Available from: https://www.who.int/publications/i/item/9789240053779

[45] Institute of Medicine. Committee for the Study on Malaria Prevention

and Control. Carpenter CC, Pearson GW, Mitchell VS, Oaks Jr SC. Malaria: obstacles and opportunities. US: National Academies Press; 1991. Available from: https://nap.nationalacademies.org/catalog/1812/malaria-obstacles-and-opportunities

[46] Al-Adhroey AH, Nor ZM, Al-Mekhlafi HM, Mahmud R. Opportunities and obstacles to the elimination of malaria from Peninsular Malaysia: Knowledge, attitudes and practices on malaria among aboriginal and rural communities. Malaria Journal. 2010;**9**:137

[47] Su XZ, Zhang C, Joy DA. Host-malaria parasite interactions and impacts on mutual evolution. Frontiers in Cellular and Infection Microbiology. 2020;**10**:587933

[48] WHO. The Global Health Observatory: WHO. 2020. Available from: https://www.who.int/data/gho/data/themes/malaria#:~:text=According%20to%20the%20World%20Malaria,again%20to%2059%20in%202020

[49] WHO. World Malaria Report 2018. Geneva: WHO; 2018

[50] Sharma S, Verma R, Yadav B, Kumar A, Rahi M, Sharma A. What India can learn from globally successful malaria elimination programmes. BMJ Global Health. 2022;7(6):1-10

[51] Global Burden of Disease Health Financing Collaborator N. Health sector spending and spending on HIV/AIDS, tuberculosis, and malaria, and development assistance for health: Progress towards Sustainable Development Goal 3. Lancet. 2020;**396**(10252):693-724

[52] Karema C, Wen S, Sidibe A, Smith JL, Gosling R, Hakizimana E, et al. History of malaria control in Rwanda: Implications for future elimination in Rwanda and other malaria-endemic countries. Malaria Journal. 2020;**19**(1):356

[53] van den Berg H, da Silva Bezerra HS, Chanda E, Al-Eryani S, Nagpal BN, Gasimov E, et al. Management of insecticides for use in disease vector control: A global survey. BMC Infectious Diseases. 2021;**21**(1):468

[54] Wilson AL, Courtenay O, Kelly-Hope LA, Scott TW, Takken W, Torr SJ, et al. The importance of vector control for the control and elimination of vector-borne diseases. PLoS Neglected Tropical Diseases. 2020;**14**(1):e0007831

[55] Mills A, Lubell Y, Hanson K. Malaria eradication: The economic, financial and institutional challenge. Malaria Journal. 2008;7(Suppl 1):S11

[56] Smith NR, Trauer JM, Gambhir M, Richards JS, Maude RJ, Keith JM, et al. Agent-based models of malaria transmission: A systematic review. Malaria Journal. 2018;**17**(1):299

[57] Cohen JM, Smith DL, Cotter C, Ward A, Yamey G, Sabot OJ, et al. Malaria resurgence: A systematic review and assessment of its causes. Malaria Journal. 2012;**11**:122

[58] Biselli R, Nisini R, Lista F, Autore A, Lastilla M, De Lorenzo G, et al. A historical review of military medical strategies for fighting infectious diseases: From battlefields to global health. Biomedicine. 2022;**10**(8)

[59] Hii J, Hustedt J, Bangs MJ. Residual malaria transmission in select countries of asia-pacific region: Old wine in a new barrel. The Journal of Infectious Diseases. 2021;**223**(12 Suppl. 2):S111-SS42

[60] Ochomo E, Chahilu M, Cook J, Kinyari T, Bayoh NM, West P, et al. Insecticide-treated nets and protection

against insecticide-resistant malaria vectors in Western Kenya. Emerging Infectious Diseases. 2017;**23**(5):758-764

[61] Ho JK, Jeevan-Raj B, Netter HJ. Hepatitis B virus (HBV) Subviral particles as protective vaccines and vaccine platforms. Viruses. 2020;**12**(2)

[62] Laurens MB. RTS,S/AS01 vaccine (Mosquirix): An overview. Human Vaccines & Immunotherapeutics. 2020;**16**(3):480-489

[63] Arora N, L CA, Pannu AK. Towards eradication of malaria: Is the WHO's RTS,S/AS01 vaccination effective enough? Risk Management in Healthcare Policy. 2021;**14**:1033-1039

[64] Editorial. Tackling poverty in tuberculosis control. Lancet. 2005;**366**(9503):2063

[65] Oxlade O, Murray M. Tuberculosis and poverty: Why are the poor at greater risk in India? PLoS One. 2012;**7**(11):e47533

[66] Li Y, Ehiri J, Tang S, Li D, Bian Y, Lin H, et al. Factors associated with patient, and diagnostic delays in Chinese TB patients: A systematic review and meta-analysis. BMC Medicine. 2013;**11**:156

[67] Storla DG, Yimer S, Bjune GA. A systematic review of delay in the diagnosis and treatment of tuberculosis. BMC Public Health. 2008;**8**:15

[68] Luca S, Mihaescu T. History of BCG vaccine. Maedica (Bucur). 2013;**8**(1):53-58

[69] Dartois VA, Rubin EJ. Anti-tuberculosis treatment strategies and drug development: Challenges and priorities. Nature Reviews. Microbiology. 2022;**20**(11):685-701. Available from: https://www.nature.com/articles/s41579-022-00731-y#citeas

[70] Matteelli A, Rendon A, Tiberi S, Al-Abri S, Voniatis C, Carvalho ACC, et al. Tuberculosis elimination: Where are we now? European Respiratory Review. 2018;**27**(148):1-15

[71] Browne SH, Umlauf A, Tucker AJ, Low J, Moser K, Gonzalez Garcia J, et al. Wirelessly observed therapy compared to directly observed therapy to confirm and support tuberculosis treatment adherence: A randomized controlled trial. PLoS Medicine. 2019;**16**(10):e1002891

[72] Fiseha D, Demissie M. Assessment of directly observed therapy (dot) following tuberculosis regimen change in Addis Ababa, Ethiopia: A qualitative study. BMC Infectious Diseases. 2015;**15**:405

[73] Wright CM, Westerkamp L, Korver S, Dobler CC. Community-based directly observed therapy (DOT) versus clinic DOT for tuberculosis: A systematic review and meta-analysis of comparative effectiveness. BMC Infectious Diseases. 2015;**15**:210

[74] Garcia JI, Mambuque E, Nguenha D, Vilanculo F, Sacoor C, Sequera VG, et al. Mortality and risk of tuberculosis among people living with HIV in whom TB was initially ruled out. Scientific Reports. 2020;**10**(1):15442

[75] Klohe K, Amuasi J, Kaducu JM, Haavardsson I, Bogatyreva E, Onarheim KH, et al. The 2017 Oslo conference report on neglected tropical diseases and emerging/re-emerging infectious diseases - Focus on populations underserved. Infectious Diseases of Poverty. 2019;**8**(1):40

[76] WHO. Ending the Neglect to Attain the Sustainable Development Goals.

A Road Map for Neglected Tropical Diseases 2021-2030. WHO; 2020. Available from: https://www.who.int/publications/i/item/9789240010352

[77] Montiel Ishino FA, Rowan C, Talham C, Villalobos K, Poudel D, Rajbhandari-Thapa J, et al. Household profiles of neglected tropical disease symptoms among children: A latent class analysis of built-environment features of Tanzanian households using the demographic and health survey. Journal of Global Health. 2022;**12**:04067

[78] Ochola EA, Karanja DMS, Elliott SJ. Local tips, global impact: Community-driven measures as avenues of promoting inclusion in the control of neglected tropical diseases: A case study in Kenya. Infectious Diseases of Poverty. 2022;**11**(1):88

[79] Pennance T, Ame SM, Amour AK, Suleiman KR, Muhsin MA, Kabole F, et al. Transmission and diversity of Schistosoma haematobium and S. bovis and their freshwater intermediate snail hosts Bulinus globosus and B. nasutus in the Zanzibar Archipelago, United Republic of Tanzania. PLoS Neglected Tropical Diseases. 2022;**16**(7):e0010585

[80] Pradhan AU, Uwishema O, Wellington J, Nisingizwe P, Thambi VD, Onyeaka CVP, et al. Challenges of addressing neglected tropical diseases amidst the COVID-19 pandemic in Africa: A case of Chagas disease. Annals of Medicine and Surgery. 2022;**81**:104414

[81] Schmidt CA, Cromwell EA, Hill E, Donkers KM, Schipp MF, Johnson KB, et al. The prevalence of onchocerciasis in Africa and Yemen, 2000-2018: A geospatial analysis. BMC Medicine. 2022;**20**(1):293

[82] Tambo E, Al-Nazawi AM. Combating the global spread of poverty-related Monkeypox outbreaks and beyond. Infectious Diseases of Poverty. 2022;**11**(1):80

[83] Ugai K, Koffi DY, Kouadio K, Yao A, Yotsu RR. Nutritional status and wound healing in patients with Mycobacterium ulcerans disease (Buruli ulcer): A pilot study from rural Cote d'Ivoire. European Journal of Dermatology. 2022;**32**(2):227-236

[84] Weld ED, Waitt C, Barnes K, Garcia BF. Twice neglected? Neglected diseases in neglected populations. British Journal of Clinical Pharmacology. 2022;**88**(2):367-373

Chapter 2

Climate Change, Conflict, and Contagion: Emerging Threats to Global Public Health

Aaron Briggs

Abstract

The present era is defined by a confluence of crises and a degree of global interconnectedness without historic precedent. A Toxic Triumvirate of climate change, conflict, and contagion have synergistically functioned to cast our collective, global public health into extreme jeopardy. The COVID-19 pandemic, War in Ukraine, and advancing climactic catastrophe have devastated our world: destabilizing nations, severing vital supply lines, and fracturing indispensable health infrastructure. All the while, *the threat of nuclear war* and the risk of devastating pandemic from emerging infectious disease (EID) grow in the unchecked wounds of low- and middle-income countries (LMIC). Nations of the Global South have been rendered super-vulnerable to the Toxic Triumvirate's effects through historic global inequity and chronically anemic international support. These "developing" nations are subject to unsustainable extremes of risk secondary to a compounding of hazard. This amplified risk is transmitted through our world *via* vibrant arteries of commerce that intimately connect us. Our world's collective health is in a state of jeopardy demanding a vigorous, equitable, and cooperative international response. To chart a course toward a safe future for our children, we must rectify the profound inequities that present our world's shared Achilles' heel and invest in the sustainable development of LMIC.

Keywords: public health, climate change, vaccine inequality, pandemic, infectious disease, climate change, inequality, transfer of hazard

1. Introduction

> *The world is entering a new danger zone, one that is more prone to shocks that can quickly knock countries off course. After navigating extraordinary challenges over the past two-and-a-half years, further extraordinary challenges lie before us...the path ahead is likely to be just as tough, if not tougher [we must] begin with a more proactive, precautionary mindset to build resilience in a more shock-prone world.*
>
> *International Monetary Fund (IMF) Director Kristalina Georgieva, 2022.*

We are at an inflection point in history. The COVID-19 pandemic has served as a wake-up call and with the climate crisis now looming, the world is experiencing its biggest shared test since the Second World War.

The United Nations (UN) Common Agenda Report, 2022.

The needle ticks 100 seconds to Midnight. The atomic scientist's hands shake as she advanced the 2020-2022 Doomsday Clock closer to Armageddon than it had ever been. The Bulletin of Atomic Scientists, established in 1945 by Albert Einstein and Manhattan Project scientists, have watched in horror as crises have grown to become confluent, mounting a compounded risk to our collective global health that is without historical precedent.

Our international body, intimately, and vibrantly connected through coursing arteries of trade and travel, has become terminally ill. A poison of inequity taints our shared bloodstream, crippling the vital international and national organ systems it touches. Disease, violence, and climatic cataclysm have battered and deluged our world with unprecedented suffering. Beneath the bullets and bombs, the temperature and water level continue to rise, and the risk of lethal pandemic brews within the unchecked wounds of the Global South.

The upper extremities in the Global North, finding themselves circumstantially above a rising water level, have attempted to further secure themselves against catastrophe. Low- and middle-income countries (LMIC), who very literally find themselves underwater, are left to struggle for survival without sustainable and effective international support. Vital organ systems of infrastructure, indispensable to curtail our ever-advancing risk, have wasted from chronically anemic funding streams, now lying unable to maintain global homeostasis. As organs fail, our shared arterial supply lines lose pressure, and the vulnerable tissues of the Global South, deprived of support and oxygen, begin to necrose. Below the water line, impoverished and traumatized communities become a gangrenous point of entry for fatal superinfection capable of disseminating through our world's circulatory system like wildfire.

At our body's beating heart, nations stand united to treat these life-threatening wounds and protect our collective health. However, their work has been stymied and paralyzed by the reluctance of wealthy, non-LMIC nations of the Global North to invest in the sustainable development and protection of the Global South. In our increasingly interconnected world, the Global North's historic strategy of self-protection and investment at the expense of LMIC has become a fool's errand [1–4].

1.1 An existential and ethical crisis

I begin by describing the role of justice in social cooperation...[presenting] the main idea of justice as fairness, a theory of justice that generalizes and carries to a higher level...the traditional conception of the social contract.

John Rawls, A Theory of Justice, 1971 (1921-2002).

If the misery of the poor be caused not by the laws of nature, but by our institutions, great is our sin.

Charles Darwin (1809-1882), Voyage of the Beagle.

The triumvirate specters of climate change, conflict and contagion haphazardly sway about our heads like Damocles' Blades. Bound in strengthened communion by morally decayed sinews of inequity, these Toxic Triumvirate have grown to present the human species with the greatest existential dilemma of its relatively brief history.

Climate change is advancing at a rapid pace and its effects have become of cataclysmic severity. Climactic upheaval ranging from sweeping fires across Europe to catastrophic floods in Africa and Southeast Asia have devastated and destabilized nations across the globe. Amidst catastrophe and resource limitation, old fault lines of conflict are becoming active, and new flashpoints are opening across the world at a dangerous and intensifying pace. The War in Ukraine has paralyzed international trade and economic growth in a world still attempting to recover from an ongoing SARS-CoV-2 (COVID-19) pandemic. Humanitarian catastrophes cripple the Global South amidst a maelstrom of conflict and climatic cataclysm. Within these concentrations of human suffering and misery, the specter of zoonotic pandemic from emerging infectious disease (EID) gathers strength. In our interconnected world, a single spark struck in a war-torn, impoverished, and destabilized corner of the globe has the potential to start an international blaze. United Nations (UN) Secretary General (SG) Antonio Guterres opened the 2022 77th Session of the United Nations General Assembly (UNGA) noting, "We are meeting during a time of great peril." The theme of the assembly was designated: A Watershed Moment: Transformative Solutions to Interlocking Challenges. The meeting was a call for international cooperation in facing the uniquely interrelated crises of climate change, war, and COVID-19, as well as the catastrophic humanitarian crises emerging in their midst.

The field of public health is entering an era of challenge and demand that is without historical precedent. The triune wraiths of contagion, climate change, and conflict, each representing an existential threat in their own right, present a confluent crisis demanding an urgent and vigorous international response.

In this chapter, I will advocate for an approach to improving and preserving global health security that leverages the power of international solidarity and sustainable development to decrease our shared risk and to help ensure a safe and habitable world for our children. The vice of inequity has shifted from being a neglected ethical responsibility to an existential imperative. The present era demands that humanity reconcile the disparities that have so marred our past, or risk succumbing to the bitter fruit of our pride & prejudice [5–9].

2. Inequality: a lethal intoxicant

> *All human beings are born free and equal in dignity and rights. They are endowed with reason and conscience and should act towards one another in a spirit of brotherhood.*
>
> *Universal Declaration of Human Rights, (UNDR) Article 1, 1948.*
>
> *There is no food. There is no medicine. The floodwaters have reached the village. Our children are sick, starving, and dying and there is nothing we can do.... *weeping**
>
> *S Sudanese Woman Interview Transcription, Al Jazeera (AJ), Oct 22, 2022.*

On December 10, 1948, the UNGA signed the United Declaration of Human Rights (UDHR) into inception, representing an important, global ethical advance. However, while nations proclaim support for the UDHR, basic rights remain unprotected across the world.

We live in an interconnected era where health and risk have become socialized and globally shared. The hazardous conditions presented by inequality anywhere reduce the safety of people everywhere. This is exemplified by the inequitable response to the COVID-19 pandemic, where critical under vaccination within the Global South has facilitated the development and circulation of COVID-19 variants that have wreaked havoc across wealthy and impoverished nations alike.

Inequity is fundamental to the persistence of COVID-19 and represents an increasingly exposed Achilles' heel for the continued recurrence of internationally paralytic pandemics. The international inequity and impoverishment that cripples nations of the Global South is not a natural phenomenon. Current global inequality has been created and maintained by specific national and international interventions, and it can be undone just the same. We enter an era where the reconciliation of international inequities must be expediently and sustainably accomplished if we are to meaningfully reduce our historic level of international risk [10–12].

2.1 One health and one risk

> *Vaccine inequity is the world's biggest obstacle to ending this pandemic and recovering from COVID-19.*
>
> *Dr. Tedros Ghebreyesus, World Health Organization (WHO) Director-General.*
>
> *Complex risks result from multiple [catastrophic] hazards occurring concurrently, and from multiple risks interacting, compounding overall risk and resulting in risk transmitting through interconnected systems and across regions.*
>
> *Intergovernmental Panel on Climate Change (IPCC) 6th Assessment Report, 2021-2022.*

The concept of One Health emerged as a solemn acknowledgment of the complexity of human health and the myriad of critical socioeconomic and environmental factors that influence it.

In 2021, the World Health Organization (WHO) formed the One Health High-Level Expert Panel (OHHLEP) to advise a multidisciplinary approach to address climate change as well as disparities in global infrastructure, agriculture, and environmental resilience.

These critical inequities pose a threat to global health with their combined effect noted to increase conditions favorable for pandemic pathogen introduction and dissemination, hereby referred to as *pathopermissive*. Because of how interconnected our global community is, the health and risk to one population is shared by all constituents of our international body [9, 13, 14].

2.2 The challenge before us

> *Contemporary global inequalities are close to early 20th-century levels, at the peak of Western imperialism.*

International Monetary Fund (IMF) World Inequality Report (WIR), 2022.

After centuries of [colonial] unreality, after having wallowed in the most outlandish phantoms... the youth of a colonized country [are forced to grow] up in an atmosphere of shot and fire...

Frantz Fanon, MD (1925-1961). Wretched of the Earth.

In this age of unprecedented and complex risk to global health, the safety of our international community will rest upon cooperative, responsive, and effective international leadership. This is an area of urgent and utmost need. Global voices including Antonio Guterres and Pope Francis have sharply criticized the failure of current national and international leadership amidst COVID-19, the War in Ukraine, and climate change.

The COVID-19 pandemic has demonstrated that one of the largest contributors of international impotence is a lack of intergovernmental coordination and a poverty of financial commitment by wealthy nations. Our current lack of intact and effective health systems in the Global South will result in critical delay of pandemic detection. The risk wrought by this disparity in health infrastructure is compounded by critical inequities in other fundamental domains including: financial resources, education, food security, essential water/sanitation/hygiene, and energy infrastructure.

The extreme concentrations of hazard and risk present in LMIC of the Global South is transmitted and disemminated among our global community through a common international circulatory system. If we are to safely navigate this perilous era, we will need to repair the wounds of the past and equip nations of the Global South with the critical infrastructure they will require to reduce the currently unsustainable levels of global risk [9, 15, 16].

2.3 Vital organs: five fundamental equalities

Imperialism leaves behind germs of rot which we must clinically detect and remove from our land [and] from our minds as well.

Frantz Fanon, MD (1925-1961). Wretched of the Earth.

We stress at the outset that addressing the challenges of the twenty first century is not feasible without significant redistribution of income and wealth inequalities.

International Monetary Fund (IMF) World Inequality Report (WIR), 2022.

The benefit of even a perfect medicine is precluded in the absence of vital organs. Likewise, sustained development can only take root in the setting of functional, essential national infrastructure. Below I will review five essential equalities that are prerequisite to the sustainable and empowered global development that must be expeditiously accomplished if we are to mitigate our present level of risk [9, 15, 16].

2.3.1 Global wealth equality

...the rules of the [international financial] game...are completely against the interests of developing countries...with debt problems, with liquidity problems, with inflation

problems, with instability, necessarily posed by this profound injustice in international financial and economic relations.

UNSG Antonio Guterres, High-Level Meeting on the Sahel, UNGA 77th Session, September 2022.

What matters [ultimately], the issue which blocks the horizon, is the need for a redistribution of wealth. Humanity will have to address this question.

Frantz Fanon, MD (1925-1961). Wretched of the Earth.

Global wealth inequality has not changed in over a century. Wealth and finance, essential for the development of any nation, are home to some of our world's most egregious disparities. The Internal Monetary Fund (IMF) published its 2022 World Inequality Report (WIR) decrying severe disparities that developmentally stymie the Global South. The report indicated that approximately 10% of the world's population is responsible for 76% of global wealth, 52% of global income, and 48% of global carbon emissions. The poorest half of our global community was found to earn only 8.5% of world wealth. Despite our stated international commitment to reconciling fundamental disparities in wealth, the inequities that cripple the Global South remain as stark as observed in 1920.

October 10, 2022: The IMF and World Bank Group (WBG) began their annual meeting in Washington, D.C. to discuss the urgent issues of global economic downturn, poverty eradication, and economic development. The summative conclusions reported as the meeting progressed are grim. The twin crises of COVID-19 and the War in Ukraine have devastated the global economy resulting in skyrocketing inflation. In the wake of systemic, economic incapacitation, national GDP has been in free-fall affecting nations of the Global South disproportionately. Nations of the Global North have also been severely impacted, with the IMF forecasting diminishing national growth and possible, global recession into 2023 [15, 17].

2.3.2 Universal energy infrastructure

If we use our fuel to get our power, we are living on our capital and exhausting it rapidly. This method is barbarous and wantonly wasteful and will have to be stopped in the interest of coming generations.

Nikola Tesla, The Wonder World To Be Created By Electricity: Manufacturer Record, 1915.

Energy has been essential for human survival from time immemorable, but it comes at a price. Western European countries have experienced significant rises in energy and cost of living as international energy infrastructure has been critically disrupted by the conflict in Ukraine.

The Global South pays a different price. Inhaled air pollutants like combustion byproducts represent a leading cause of global morbidity and mortality estimated to be responsible for more than 10 million excess deaths each year. This suffering is disproportionately concentrated in LMIC whose infrastructural development and energy transition have been curtailed by international intervention and negligence.

The 1970s brought an American-led end to the Post-WWII Breton Woods International Economic System that had previously constrained the corporate flow of capital. In its place, a neoliberal, political-economic policy permitting ruthless corporate expansion and exploitation further deepened our global inequities. The Global North, having stumbled through the perils of industrial revolution at catastrophic cost to domestic labor workforce and the international poor, begin to power a transition to improved forms of energy by exporting upscaled, dangerous, and crude manufacturing processes to LMIC. The pressure to exploit LMIC as regions of manufacture due to lax labor and environmental regulation led to a critical *shift of environmental hazard* from the Global North to South.

Currently, approximately 50% of the world's population lack access to improved energy infrastructure and are dependent on solid fuels, which result in substantial increases in exposure to combustion's mediators of disease.

When energy infrastructure fails, cataclysm can become a catastrophe. Climate change and conflict have taken devastating tolls on the infrastructural integrity of nations across the world. Ukraine, following Russian shelling in early October, had lost 40% of its energy infrastructure resulting in sweeping outages and their pathologic sequela such as loss of access to clean drinking water and failure of sanitation resources [9, 18, 19].

2.3.3 Universal food security

> *The water is dirty and the trip to get it is dangerous. I have to leave my children and by the time I arrive home it is dark. Today I do not know what my children will eat. Everyone has been affected by the drought. Our rains have failed, our children are not eating and going to sleep hungry. We need help we are hungry and cannot survive like this.*
>
> *Kenyan Woman, Interviewed AJ Oct 2022, Translated into English and Transcribed.*
>
> *Conflict, COVID, the climate crisis and rising costs have combined in 2022 to create jeopardy for up to 828 million hungry people across the world.... While needs are sky-high, resources have hit rock bottom.*
>
> *World Food Programme (WFP).*

We have lost progress in the fight against global hunger. In 2022 the World Food Programme (WFP) declared a global food crisis, noting this to be a year of unprecedented food insecurity. The UN/WHO 2022 State of Food Security and Nutrition in the World Report described a deepening inequity in access to food that is heavily impacting the Global South. As of the late 2022 writing of this chapter, the African Horn and Eastern Africa are experiencing drought-induced famine with affected nations demonstrating concerning rises in child malnutrition. Last year in flood-stricken Nigeria, the WFP announced that it would have to reduce food support by 50% due to funding limitations. At a time when international need has peaked, the anemic support from the Global North that has become the historic norm must change. Across the world, malnutrition is acting to weaken immune systems in the regions where outbreak risk is the highest. To leave nations to succumb beneath conflict, climactic catastrophe, and hunger represents both a reckless jeopardization of our collective health and an absysmal ethical failure [20, 21].

2.3.4 Universal water, sanitation, and hygiene (WASH) infrastructure

Half of healthcare facilities globally lack basic hygiene services. 1 in 3 people globally do not have access to clean drinking water.

WHO, United Nations International Children's Emergency Fund (UNICEF) Report and Press Release: 2019, 2022.

Countries must double their efforts on sanitation or we will not reach universal access by 2030. If countries fail to step up efforts on sanitation, safe water and hygiene, we will continue to live with diseases that should have been long ago consigned to the history books:

Dr. Maria Neira, WHO Director, Department of Public Health, Environmental and Social Determinants of Health.

The WHO and United Nations International Children's Fund (UNICEF) Joint Monitoring Program (JMP) has been monitoring global access to water, sanitation, and hygiene (WASH) infrastructure since its inception in 1990. Currently, 2.1 billion people lack access to safe drinking water and 4.5 billion people lack sanitation. Approximately 800 children die from preventable diarrheal illness every day because of this. Nearly all of the nations still requiring WASH infrastructure are located on the African continent. The lack of WASH infrastructure affects much more than health. Clean water and sanitation are essential for the development of children, economies, and nations. As such, this inequity represents a key barrier to the sustainable global development we will need to improve our collective safety. The UNICEF 2016-2030 WASH framework is designed to rectify this inequity with the goal of achieving universal and equitable access to safe water, sanitation, and hygiene by 2030. However, as with many efforts toward equity, the UNICEF WASH initiative has been critically frustrated by chronically anemic financial support from wealthy nations of the Global North [22, 23].

2.3.5 Universal national health infrastructure

In Africa, most people are born, live, and die without leaving a trace in the official record.

Don de Savigny, Tanzania Essential Health Interventions Project.

It has long been recognized that a malarious community is an impoverished community.

T. H. Weller, Nobel Laureate in Medicine, 1958.

On Saturday night the doctor called me said my daughter is critical. All her organs are damaged, her brain, her heart and her eyes. On Sunday morning she had heart failure and died in my lap. The government needs to investigate this and come up with solutions. I do not want any mother to feel what I felt. I've lost my baby.

Indonesian woman, Interviewed AJ Oct 22, 2022, Translated into English and transcribed.

In early October 2022, 70 children passed from acute kidney failure in the Gambia. The culprit was found to be tainted cough syrup shipped from an Indian pharmaceutical company. In the late 2022 final drafting of this chapter, more than 130 children were reported to have passed from acute kidney illness secondary to cough syrup in Indonesia and the case count is rising.

Vulnerable children are said to be "an infection away from catastrophe" and not even their medicine is safe. Global inequity in health infrastructure takes an immeasurable toll on LMIC. Preventable diseases of poverty shackle the economies of the Global South, while waves of outbreak from Ebola to COVID batter nations like storm surges.

Global equality in health infrastructure is the cornerstone of our defense against pandemic. In order for deadly pathogen to be effectively identified and contained within the region of introduction, there must be essential national health infrastructure in place. In its absence, such as in the 2014 Ebola Epidemic, outbreaks are able to spread unmitigated and undetected like wildfire. Functional national health infrastructure is also imperative to the control of the preventable diseases of poverty that disproportionately take their toll on the youngest generations—crippling the capacity of affected nations to develop.

Recent research on the health infrastructure of LMIC has articulated three consistent features found in health systems of the Global South: insufficient resources, weak state effective capacity, and high burden of disease. As their internal capability for development has been critically impaired, nations of the Global South will require significant and expedient international investment to kick-start the establishment of functional and sustainable civil infrastructure and healthcare systems. Universal health infrastructure will be fundamental to our global safety as effective, local pandemic preparedness and disaster response will require organized and decisive national action in order to control fires at their source [24–28].

2.4 A road to sustainable development

> *Evidence of observed impacts, projected risks, levels and trends in vulnerability, and adaptation limits demonstrate that worldwide [catastrophically] resilient development action is more urgent than previously assessed.*
>
> *IPCC 6th Assessment, 2022.*

The reviewed dilemmas of inequality represent recognized global emergencies to which the UN, WHO, and other international actors have responded. In the year 2000, the Millennium Development Goals (MDG) were designated by the UN. These eight goals represented key global disparities to be addressed through an internationally cooperative response.

The Sustainable Development Goals (SDG) were designated in 2015, immediately in succession of the MDG. The SDG represent an enhanced set of aims incorporating lessons learned from the prior MDG and distinguish themselves in their focus on sustainability. Chronic inequity has rendered nations of the Global South uniquely disempowered to affect their own development with many prior interventions in the Global South having been reactive, superficial, and unsustainable. Nations of the Global South must be released from poverty, debt, disease and violence, and empowered to develop and build the capacity necessary to weather the storms to come. In our present world, the health of our global community depends on the health of its constituents. The watershed of development proposed in the SDG will likely generate a positive feedback cycle as more and more citizens of the world are released from inequity's shackles and empowered to contribute to the building of a cooperative, safe, and more resilient tomorrow [1, 3, 9, 29, 30].

3. Climate change: the crisis to define an era

> *I have just returned from Pakistan, where I looked through a window into the future. A future of permanent and ubiquitous climate chaos on an unimaginable scale: Devastating loss of life, enormous human suffering, and massive damage to infrastructure and livelihoods. It is simply heartbreaking.*
>
> *No picture can convey the scope of this catastrophe.... What is happening in Pakistan demonstrates the sheer inadequacy of the global response to the climate crisis, and the betrayal and injustice at the heart of it.*
>
> *UNSG Antonio Guterres, 77th UNGA, Opening Press Conference. September 2022.*

October 2022: Approximately one-third of Pakistan is flooded, about 1.6 million children face malnutrition, and UNICEF has received only 30% of the funds necessary to mount the required response. Amidst the stagnant waters and rubble, reports indicate that waterborne and respiratory diseases are spreading.

Climate change has become the defining issue of our time. Such was the consensus among international leaders at the 77th UNGA High-Level Meeting on Climate Change. During the meeting, LMIC leaders noted concern at the faltering pace of climate adaptation and mitigation, calling for increased investment and accountability from the wealthy nations largely responsible the climate crisis.

The Intergovernmental Panel on Climate Change (IPCC) is the UN organization charged with empirically assessing climate change on Earth. The IPCC includes experts from around the world and is recognized as the foremost international scientific authority on climate change. In 2022, the body published its sixth assessment, emphasizing the existential severity of the crisis we are facing and decrying the lack of commitment from the Global North in rectifying the present catastrophe and preventing terminal escalation of cascading climatic processes.

Thus far, the Earth has warmed approximately 1.09°C above the pre-industrial temperatures noted prior to the turn of the twentieth century. The IPCC designated a critical threshold of 1.5°C increase above pre-industrial temperatures as being associated with significant increases in multiple climactic hazards with substantial projected loss of life and infrastructure. The Paris Agreement, the global rallying point for cooperative climate action, recognizes this threshold. However, our efforts have not been sufficient to curtail our advance—this is largely due to a lack of financial commitment from wealthy nations. The IPCC predicts a 50% chance of the Earth warming to 1.5°C within the next 20 years if the current trajectory is continued. As climate change and its aftershocks wreak havoc on international trade and agriculture, erode national economies, and devastate infrastructure, people suffer.

In the Global North, rising housing prices and anger over climate inaction motivates tens of thousands to march through their streets. For their counterparts in the Global South, the impact of climate change is measured in blood [3, 8, 9, 31].

3.1 The impacts of climate change

> *Climate change is a threat to human well-being and planetary health....increases in frequency and intensity of extremes have reduced food and water security hindering efforts to meet Sustainable Development Goals.*
>
> *IPCC 6th Assessment, 2022.*
>
> *Diseases have attacked us because we are all still standing in the water...*
>
> *Pakistani man, Interviewed AJ Oct 22, 2022, Translated into English and transcribed.*

Drought has suffocated the African Sahel and Horn leading to a vicious cycle of hunger conflict, and destabilization. Amidst the compounded suffering and concentrated misery, African leaders ask for their continent not to be forgotten.

Climate change is an active force of destabilization in our world that has wreaked havoc on the most vulnerable and its effects are accelerating. Unprecedented and devastating extremes of weather have been observed across the globe at increasing rates. Amplified monsoon seasons bring devastating flooding to Pakistan, and high-powered hurricanes batter the Caribbean and Central America. With floodwater and torrential wind come chaos, loss, trauma, destruction of livelihood, and the disruption of essential national infrastructure. In this way, climate change functions not only to injure humanity in its own right, but also functions to create conditions pathopermissive to violence and disease [3, 8, 9, 32].

3.2 Climate change risks

> *Climate change impact and risk are becoming increasingly complex and difficult to manage. Multiple climate hazards will occur simultaneously, and multiple climactic and non-climactic risks will interact, resulting in compounding overall risk...*
>
> *IPCC 6th Assessment Report, 2022.*

Climate change distinguishes itself from its Triumvirate counterparts in that it is a significant amplifier of risk. War-torn nations and refugee populations have always represented extreme vulnerability. Climate change adds to this risk in a globally pervasive and devastating manner that is without historical precedent.

Climate change's ability to exacerbate the inequities that multiply its catastrophic impact among LMIC is why it must be designated a priority threat to global health and safety. Numerous LMIC, rendered historically vulnerable to climactic upheaval by years of inequity, lie devastated and left to recover with insufficient resources. Beneath climactic calamity and fog of war, malnourished immune-compromised refugee populations journey through stagnant, mosquito-laced waters to huddle together in unsanitary, makeshift refugee camps. The specter of disease closely accompanies them, gaining strength amidst the chaos and trauma that riddle the Global South.

To allow historically maimed LMIC nations to struggle for survival in the midst of devastating cataclysm and conflict is to permit the compounding, superaddition of risk factors that will existentially threaten the health of our international community.

Climate change has tilled through the Global South uprooting populations and fracturing infrastructure—all the while providing increasingly fertile ground for conflict and deadly disease [3, 8, 9, 33].

3.3 Climate resilient development

> *Any further delay in concerted anticipatory global action on adaptation and mitigation will miss a brief and rapidly closing window of opportunity to secure a livable and sustainable future for all.*
>
> *IPCC 6th Assessment Report, 2022*

December 12, 2015: The Paris Climate Agreement was signed into inception and adopted by 196 nations. The agreement provided succession to the Kyoto Climate Protocol signed in 1997 and officially entering into force on November 4, 2016. The Paris Agreement is legally binding and represents the current international effort to address climate change. The two main pillars of its response are adaptation and mitigation.

Adaptation involves the active protection of vulnerable communities now—increasing current resilience against catastrophe. Mitigation works to provide sustained protection in the future *via* the reversal of the vicious cycles that are driving the process. The Paris Agreement noted a goal of curbing global pre-industrial temperature increase below 1.5°C in recognition of the significantly increased hazard predicted by the IPCC beyond this threshold.

While the Paris Treaty provided a rejuvenating burst to climate change response, the battle against climate change has since stalled amidst a trend of waning investment from wealthy nations. While significant contributions have occurred, most funds have been dedicated to mitigation with little investment directed toward providing immediate, adaptive support for the LMIC nations who are being deluged and drowned beneath reiterant climatic catastrophes. Nations of the Global South must be expediently released from the shackles of poverty and hunger that constrain their national growth and must be assisted in the construction of resilient, essential infrastructure that will be fundamental to the empowered and sustained development of LMIC nations. With the five inequities reviewed addressed at minimum, adaptive measures can be more effectively and sustainably implemented, and nations of the Global South can be given freedom to undertake necessary, self-guided development [3, 8, 9, 34].

4. Geopolitical tension and state conflict

> *We came very, very close [to nuclear war,] closer than we knew at the time.*
>
> *Robert McNamara, late US Secretary of Defense*
>
> *This was not only the most dangerous moment of the Cold War. It was the most dangerous moment in human history.*
>
> *Arthur M. Schlesinger Jr., late advisor to President John F Kennedy*

October 27, 1962: Cuban Missile Crisis. A Soviet Foxtrot Class B59 submarine carrying a nuclear payload slipped through the Caribbean off the coast of Cuba.

Onboard was one Vasily Arkhipov (1926–1998), a then officer in the Soviet navy hailing from a humble background. An American destroyer had identified the vessel on sonar and began dropping depth charges. In response, the submarine was forced to dive to a depth from which Soviet radio communication could not be received. Amidst the subaquatic explosions, leaking water, and rising carbon dioxide levels, the ship's captain and political officers noted that a war had likely started, and the submarine should fire its nuclear payload. Vasily Arkhipov, then known and admired for prior demonstrations of courage, denied the order. He is widely recognized for his decisive, maverick action that saved the world from thermonuclear war. Until now, this has been regarded as the closest humanity has been to annihilation.

Six decades have passed and we continue to live beneath an ever-growing shadow of nuclear war. Thermonuclear Armageddon has been averted by the chance, heroic action of a single individual. This is no model for sustainability and the odds say that if we continue to roll the dice as we have, we will run up against our number. For all intents and purposes, in 1962, we already had [35–37].

4.1 100 seconds to midnight

> *We can hear once again the rattling of nuclear sabres...The idea that any country could fight and win a nuclear war is deranged. Any use of a nuclear weapon would incite a humanitarian Armageddon. We need to step back.*
>
> *UN General Assembly 2022 UNSG Antonio Guterres on Nuclear Disarmament*

> *I know not with what weapons world war III will be fought. But world war IV will be fought with sticks and stones.*
>
> *Albert Einstein*

We live in an unstable world precariously balanced on a razor's edge between peace and catastrophic war. The introduction of weapons of mass destruction (WMD) with the nuclear bomb in 1945 marked a pivotal turning point in human history. We had advanced technologically to a degree where we now held keys to our own destruction. The Bulletin of Atomic Scientists was established by Albert Einstein in solemn recognition of this. The risk and reach of conflict had critically extended from regionally limited devastation to now represent an existential, global threat. There are no winners in a nuclear conflict, it will be universally catastrophic.

From 1945 onward, the world has lived in the shadow of nuclear annihilation, and the Bulletin has closely watched. The Doomsday Clock was wound into motion in 1947 with the newly nuclear armed world set at 7 minutes to apocalyptic midnight. The Cold War Period brought the world to the brink of nuclear annihilation multiple times and advanced the clock to 2 minutes to midnight. This would be the closest humanity would dance with annihilation until 2018 when the mounting hazards of climate change and conflict returned the world to a Cold War level of risk. The progression of these crises and the introduction of a devastating, global pandemic prompted the Bulletin to advance the Clock to 100 seconds to midnight in 2020. This is closest humanity has come to existential catastrophe and the clock has remained fixed "on doom's doorstep" ever since [4, 38].

4.2 Global arms control

> *Nuclear weapons are the most destructive power ever created. They offer no security — just carnage and chaos. Their elimination would be the greatest gift we could bestow on future generations.*
>
> *UNGA 77th Session 2022: UNSG Antonio Guterres on Nuclear Weapons.*
>
> *The world is currently at a height of nuclear Armageddon risk not seen in 60 years.*
>
> *Joseph Biden, 46th President of the United States.*

June 2001: A working group with the John's Hopkins Center for Health Security convene in Washington, D.C. for an exercise amidst growing concerns of WMD mass casualty events. The operation was called *Dark Winter*, and it was a modeled simulation of a bioterror attack on the United States. In the scenario, a smallpox outbreak was unable to be contained and spread through the continental United States like wildfire. The operation noted a concerning lack of surge capacity and preparation within the American health, pharmaceutical, and vaccine systems. *Dark Winter's* conclusion predicted massive civilian casualties, a breakdown in essential institutions, loss of confidence in the government, and extreme civil unrest. This noted vulnerability began a series of regular pandemic exercises that have continued to 2019. In June of this year, President Vladamir Putin of Russia and Alex Lukashenjo of Belarus agree to the deployment of Russian short-range nuclear-capable missiles in Belarus. As geopolitical tensions rise and exacerbating risk factors wreak havoc across the world, now more than ever, effective global arms control is needed if we are to safeguard our international community.

Four of the fundamental global arms treaties are the: Non-Proliferation Treaty (NPT), the New START treaty, The Chemical Weapons Convention (CWC), and The Biological Weapons Convention (BWC). Each of these international agreements found their inception in the latter half of the twentieth century when concern for terminal catastrophe from WMD had reached a crescendo. However, despite these efforts, nuclear arsenal stockpiles remain high, and a number of nations have raised concerns regarding active engagement in biologic and chemical warfare research. The frustrated progress of global arms control has been grossly contributed to by a lack of: funding, member state cooperation, and verification/enforcement capacity.

In response to the persistent and extreme hazard from WMD, the United Nations adopted and ratified the Treaty on the Prohibition of Nuclear Weapons (TPNW) in 2020. The treaty became active January of 2021. However, reminiscent of past stumbling blocks, 69 nations abstained from becoming party; pertinently: all nuclear-armed world powers and nearly all NATO member states. The new arms control treaty provides comprehensive restrictions to nuclear weapon: development, testing, stockpile, transfer, stationing, and use. The ultimate goal of the TPNW is to achieve total nuclear arms elimination.

Superpower reluctance to ratify and commit to the TPNW renders the NPT the only binding treaty signed by the world's nuclear armed states. In the fall of 2022, UNSG Antonio Guterres convened a meeting of United Nations member states to review and re-commit to the NPT. However, after 4 weeks of intense negotiation, a consensus was unable to be reached—chiefly because of unilateral and discordant action taken by nuclear powers.

A review of major arms treaties demonstrates a concerning trend of waning international commitment to a sustainable and peaceful future. The United States, China, and Russia have been undertaking nuclear modernization and expansion efforts, while new arms races have started regarding emerging hypersonic and anti-satellite missile technology. However, some positive progress has been made and can be celebrated.

The American and Russian Federation New START arms reduction treaty's extension in 2021 marked a small but important step in movement toward a goal of disarmament. Since their inception, nuclear weapons have represented a ticking time bomb that have pushed humanity to the brink of annihilation on more than one occasion. We may not get another chance [4, 39–44].

4.3 The War in Ukraine

> *The idea of nuclear conflict, once unthinkable, has become a subject of debate. The vulnerable are suffering most. There is only one way to end the suffering in Ukraine and that is by ending the war.*
>
> *UN General Assembly 2022: UNSG Antonio Guterres: UN Security Council High-Level Debate on Ukraine.*

As of the final drafting of this chapter, 40% of Ukrainian energy infrastructure has been damaged by targeted Russian missile strikes and the entire country is being affected by rolling blackouts. Amidst a coming winter, Ukrainians are being directed to stockpile clean water and warm clothes.

The War in Ukraine is testament to how intimately interconnected our world is. Russia's invasion of Ukraine has reaped devastating tolls on Ukraine's population and infrastructure. Europe and the world continue to live beneath the shadow of nuclear catastrophe as tensions mount between world powers and Ukraine's Zaporizhzhia Nuclear Power Plant sustains collateral damage from the conflict.

However, thus far, some of the most devastating global effects from the conflict in Ukraine originated not from bullets or bombs, but from a critical snare of the global supply chain. The conflict has thus far pushed millions into extremes of poverty, significantly exacerbated the risk of famine, and reversed years of developmental progress.

SG Guterres and the UN quickly noted an emergency as Ukraine's grain exports plummeted following Russia's invasion. The War in Ukraine resulted in a critical disruption of global food supply that casts many impoverished regions into deeper risk of famine. The Black Sea Grain Initiative, brokered by Turkiye and the United Nations, provides an example of a successful, expeditious, and relatively equitable international response to emergency.

The disruption of the international energy supply chain prompted a global energy crisis. Nations in the Global North and South have endured significant collateral damage including: economic downturn, escalating inflation, rising costs of energy and food, internal destabilization, and escalating geopolitical tension. The impacts of war are unevenly distributed with impoverished nations rendered super-vulnerable to destabilizing collateral forces spinning off from regional and international conflicts [45, 46].

4.4 Global trends in conflict

> *Insecurity and political instability in the Sahel continue to make an already catastrophic humanitarian situation even worse. In some regions, States have totally lost*

access to their populations. Non-State armed groups are tightening their deadly grip over the region...Indiscriminate violence continues to kill and injure thousands of innocent civilians, while forcing millions of others to flee their homes.

UN General Assembly 2022: UNSG Antonio Guterres: High Level Meeting on the Sahel.

The tribal fighting has killed at least 200, and more than 200 others have been injured. In the first assessment there are 2004 families with children in 4 schools. The displacement has been massive and these displaced are now in schools in large groups. These habitats are not fit to be camps and lack the needed medical supplies. There are a lot of complications and we cannot handle the situation. The flow of displaced is growing and we are calling on aid organizations and friendly countries to send the necessary aid.

Sudanese Minister of Social Welfare, Interviewed AJ Oct 2022, Translated into English and transcribed.

October 2022: An attach on a Somali hotel by Al Shebab kills nine innocents and wounts more while interstate violence in Sudan's Blue Nile State has filled hospitals past capacity with wounded. The fighting has resulted in significant displacement that has forced fleeing refugees into crowded, unsanitary conditions. This represents a trend of irregular/asymmetric violence that has torn apart nations of the Global South for decades.

Conflict is grossly divided into two major types: interstate conflict and intrastate conflict. Wars between nations have decreased in frequency since the end of World War II. However, intrastate conflicts have increased in frequency at an accelerating rate, particularly with the Global South. Since 2010, there has been a noted threefold increase in major civil war frequency, a sixfold increase in conflict mortality, and an approximately 60% rate of conflict recurrence.

This internal, irregular violence has been tearing nations of the Global South apart taking an especially heavy toll on the African continent. At the 2022 General Assembly, SG Guterres held a High-Level Meeting on the Sahel. During the meeting, SG Guterres expressed significant concern over the progressing risk and complexity of the Sahel's geopolitical situation as climate disruption, energy crisis, famine, and crippling impoverishment destabilize nations and spark intrastate violence. The increasingly recalcitrant and intractable nature of conflict is amplified by this noted uptick in complexity with many intrastate conflicts now proving less responsive to traditional political and diplomatic measures of resolution [33, 47, 48].

4.5 The impacts of conflict

Armed conflict not only directly interferes with [Sustainable Development Goal]16, it negatively affects key targets of the entire UN sustainable development agenda.... Going well beyond direct death and physical destruction...consequences [of conflict] involve devastating long-term damage to social networks, human capital and trust in institutions that reinforce each other in powerful ways through perpetuation of violence and out-migration.

Cederman et al, 2018.

Conflict takes a heavy toll. The acute human morbidity and mortality are the most immediate and readily seen impacts of conflict. However, the aftershocks of suffering that ripple through shattered national infrastructure prove equally devastating.

The ongoing Yemeni Civil War can prove instructive regarding the compounded risk levied on populations of the Global South. The devastation of Yemen's water and sanitation infrastructure by conflict produced widespread, unsanitary, and biologically hazardous conditions. The addition of unseasonal and significant rainfall and flooding to this caustic mixture resulted in the exposure of a chronically malnournished war-torn population to a compounded infectious disease risk. This interaction of complex biologic risk with extremes of vulnerability facilitated what would become the worst cholera epidemic in modern history.

In the case of the ongoing Civil War in Syria, more than half of the nation's population has been displaced and catastrophic damage has been done to over half of essential Syrian medical, educational, and energy infrastructure. This disruption in essential infrastructure has rendered the nation's chronically war-torn resident population especially vulnerable to climatic and contagious risk resulting in excess morbidity and mortality and a decline in Syrian life expectancy by 5 years. Population displacement from concurrent crises has caused significant increased in migrant populations resulting in a strain and fracture of critically underpowered international and national refugee support networks. This ultimately exposes exceptionally vulnerable, migrant populations to extremes of risk resulting in tragic loss of life. Standing as grim testament to this, the Mediterranean Sea has slowly become a graveyard to many migrants fleeing conflict and catastrophe.

In 2022, global inflation rose to 8.8%. The IMF cites the War in Ukraine and the COVID-19 pandemic as key contributors to the global financial crisis. While both Global North and South have experienced economic impact, LMIC have borne the brunt of the injury. In their annual meeting last year, the IMF and World Bank Group expressed concern double-digit rates of inflation which have impacted 40% of countries in sub-Saharan Africa—critically impairing essential national development and providing fertile soil for seeds of conflict and disease to take root [1, 15, 33, 49].

4.6 A road to peace

> *Peace is the most important economic policy tool right now.*
>
> *Nadia Calvino, IMF Chair and Spanish Vice President.*
>
> *Without eliminating nuclear weapons, there can be no peace. There can be no trust. And there can be no sustainable future.*
>
> *UNSG Guterres.*

An overabundance of military spending and a lack of investment in sustainable, global development are actively contributing to global risk. Sustainable, global peace will require a significant shift in national priority and finance away from defense spending. Weapons must be exchanged for plowshares and soldiering must bow to solidarity. The volatile, root causes of conflict will need to be tilled up from the soil of LMIC in the Global South to make way for the sustainable development that will need to occur if we are to effectively safeguard our collective, global health security. The mechanisms to affect this development have been defined and set into motion, the lacking component has been fuel and international investment. In this dilemma, military budget reduction may provide a parsimonious and elegant way to power peace through disarmament. In addition to a treaty representing a new global commitment to disarmament, the United Nations brought *Our Common Agenda* into inception in 2020 at the 75th General Assembly. *Our Common Agenda* outlines and underscores the goals we must work to achieve in order to provide our younger generation with a safer tomorrow. The Human species has held fire in our hands for more than half a century, if we continue along this path, it is a matter of time until we are burned [2, 4, 50].

5. Contagion: the curse of inequality

> *For there can now no longer be any doubt that such an epidemic dissemination of typhus had only been possible under the wretched conditions of life that poverty...had created.*
>
> *Dr. Rudolf Virchow, 'Father of Modern Pathology.' 1848.*

Infectious disease has long been an intimate enemy of humanity. The flea vector-borne Bubonic Plague, H1N1 Influenza pandemic of 1918, and ongoing AIDS and COVID-19 pandemics offer humbling testament to human society's unique vulnerability to this curse. Contagion distinguishes itself among the Toxic Triumvirate in its long understood and inextricable relationship with conditions of poverty and inequity.

In the mid-nineteenth century, a young Dr. Rudolf Virchow was dispatched from the Prussian Ministry of Health to investigate a typhus epidemic that had been reported in the city of Upper Silesia. The dawn of the Industrial Revolution in the Global North resulted in a trend of urbanization that quickly exceeded the infrastructural carrying capacity of early cities. Crowded living conditions, poor air quality, and lack of sanitation provided conditions ideal for the spread of early urban diseases such as cholera and epidemic typhus.

Dr. Virchow was struck by the abysmal conditions of impoverishment and misery he observed among the urban poor of Upper Silesia. In his *Report on the Typhus Epidemic in Upper Silesia*, Dr. Virchow inferred that it was precisely these "adverse climactic conditions which contributed to the failure of [Upper Silesia's] crops and to the sickness of its bodies." Six years before an English anesthesiologist would begin a famous investigation of cholera in London, Dr. Virchow concluded his seminal report relating poverty and disease noting:

> *If these conditions [of poverty] were removed, I am sure that epidemic typhus would not recur. Whosoever wishes to learn from history will find many examples.*

In nineteenth century Prussia and throughout human history, contagious outbreaks have demonstrated themselves to be exquisitely socially and environmentally. The impoverished, unsanitary, and environmentally unstable conditions that plague the LMIC represent a dangerous compounding of biologic hazard. Within the growing urban-slums of the Global South, vulnerable populations are exposed to extremes of infectious disease risk that are transmitted and shared across our international community through international trade and travel. In our increasingly interconnected world, the risk endured by one population is shared by all [51–54].

5.1 Diseases of poverty: the poor man's burden

> *Poverty has been inextricably linked with infectious diseases since antiquity. Poverty, acting through non-genetic heritable principles, has transformed infectious diseases into "inheritable" conditions.*
>
> *Hansen and Paintsil, 2016*

> *Over the last 2 years, the multiple and overlapping crises that have rocked the world have...knocked back the global response to the AIDS pandemic. The new data revealed in this report are frightening: progress has been faltering, resources have been shrinking, and inequalities have been widening. Insufficient investment and action are putting all of us in danger: we face millions of AIDS-related deaths and millions of new HIV infections if we continue on our current trajectory. We can end AIDS by 2030. But the curve will not bend itself. We have to pull it down.*
>
> *UNAIDS Global AIDS Update, 2022.*

Every 2 minutes a child dies of malaria. Infectious Diseases of Poverty (IDoP) are estimated to take 14 million lives annually with children disproportionately impacted. In this way, the young generations of the Global South who will be faced with unprecedented challenge are crippled at the outstart by preventable/treatable IDoP. The infections that unnecessarily curse the world's most vulnerable are myriad, but malaria, tuberculosis (TB), and HIV have proven exceptionally devastating. This apty named, "Unholy Trinity," acting in concert with diarrheal illness and Neglected Tropical Disease (NTD), have plagued Global South for decades—devastating populations, crippling economies, and paralyzing critical development.

Malaria is a preventable illness that has been successfully eradicated from many regions of the globe. In 2020, the WHO estimated there to be 241 million cases of malaria worldwide with 627,000 total deaths. The African continent is home to 95% of malaria cases and 96% of malaria deaths—80% of which are children under 5 years old. The WHO global malaria strategy is designed to achieve 90% reduction in cases and deaths by 2030, but progress has slowed. While COVID-19 caused significant disruption to health systems and medical care across the world, some significant advances in malaria control have been achieved and retained. These include the recent introduction of a vaccine for malaria and the historic reduction in annual childhood malaria mortality from 900,000 deaths in 2000, to approximately 650,000 in 2019. Insecticide-treated bed nets were credited with being responsible for approximately 68% of the cases averted. Malaria is a treatable and eradicable disease that has been successfully banished from many nations of the Global North. It is time the Global South is released from this burden as well.

In 2021, one child died of AIDS-related causes every minute. The Joint United Nations Programme on HIV/AIDS (UNAIDS) reported 38 million people living with HIV and 650,000 AIDS-related deaths in 2021. The majority of deaths occur in children who comprise 4% of people living with HIV but 15% of age-related deaths. In 2021, an estimated 53% children living with HIV lacked access to HIV treatment. UNAIDS reports that the lion's share of HIV incidence, morbidity, mortality, and lack of treatment access is concentrated among key vulnerable global populations. Disruptions in health infrastructure by COVID-19 caused a significant loss of global progress in the battle to control AIDS with many countries experiencing increasing incidence rates. Inequity in treatment has grown as international AIDS support has fallen by 57% over the past decade with UNAIDS calling for renewed vigor and attention to be given to reducing disparities in global HIV/AIDS treatment and outcome.

Tuberculosis (TB) is a curable and preventable disease, and the second leading infectious cause of death worldwide. It exists in a viciously synergistic relationship with HIV's immunosuppression and is led only by COVID-19 in global infectious disease (ID) mortality. LMIC account for 98% of reported TB cases with countries such as India, Indonesia, Pakistan, Nigeria, and Bangladesh claiming some of the highest TB prevalence worldwide. As with the global AIDS response, international funding has been declining over time, falling 8.7% between 2019 and 2020. The UN has committed to ending the TB epidemic by 2030; however, if we are to reach this goal, channels of support must be bolstered significantly [55–59].

5.2 COVID-19: a grim teacher

> *The COVID-19 pandemic rightly has absorbed the world's attention, given its demonstrated ability to sicken and kill millions...And yet, what the world has experienced during this pandemic is nowhere close to a worst-case scenario.*
>
> *Bulletin of Atomic Scientists, 2022 Doomsday Clock Statements.*

Even a perfect medicine will be rendered inert when given in solution with inequity. This has been a public health lesson expressed ad nauseam by the cyclic, zoonotic pandemics that have become an unnecessary part of our reality. AIDS, MERS, SARS, Ebola, and now COVID-19 outbreaks/pandemics reiterantly wreaked havoc across the globe, becoming increasingly economically and sociopolitically devastating over time.

Over the past 2 years, COVID-19 has infected 767 million and killed 6.9 million, with the highest rates of excess death observed in LMIC [60]. COVID-19 crippled the global economy acting in tandem with the War in Ukraine to cause skyrocketing inflation and declining rates of national economic growth that have paralyzed or reversed developmental progress.

Both COVID-19 and non-COVID-19 zoonotic pandemics continue to represent an extreme global risk. Currently, the UN and WHO estimate that only 34% of low-income country populations have been vaccinated against COVID-19. The pandemic's persistence is owed in part to COVID-19's consistent exploitation of the vulnerabilities inherent to undervaccinated populations. One manifestation of this can be found in the mutated viral variants that develop in the shadows of vaccination. These mutant strains have continued to fuel the pandemic's slow-burn course toward global and regional endemicity [4, 53, 54, 61–63].

5.3 Emerging diseases and pandemic risk

> *The world has [long] witnessed how global travel, trade, urbanization, and environmental degradation can fuel the emergence and spread of infectious disease threats.*
>
> *Nuclear Threat Initiative, 2021.*

October 2022: Pakistan remains devastated from atypical monsoon flooding, which inundated one-third of the country. Reports from the ground describe increasing rates of waterborne illness and respiratory infection with maternal and fetal mortality rising significantly.

Emerging infectious diseases (EID) are infectious diseases to which we are naïve either because we have not met them, or because the disease we used to know has changed character physically, spatially, or biologically.

EID are comprised mostly of zoonotic pathogen such as coronaviruses, hemorrhagic fever viruses, and avian/porcine-derived influenza viruses, and represent an ever-growing threat to global public health. Over the past three decades, outbreaks of EID have been noted to increase in frequency—this disproportionately occurring within impoverished nations of the Global South. The increasing rate of emergence has been contributed to by a myriad of factors including: global warming, environmental change, dangerous animal husbandry practices and growing antimicrobial resistance. Underregulated microbiologic gain-of-function research represents a significant and growing hazard overall contributing to a historically unprecedented level of pandemic risk.

Avian influenza viruses, such as H5N1, naturally circulate among waterfowl in which they evoke a limited, mild upper respiratory inflammatory response upon initial infection. These viruses have the potential to be transmitted to chickens, pigs, and humans in whom they can elicit a much more severe and lethal inflammatory response. Of particular concern are recently detected, highly virulent avian viruses such as H5N9, which have caused numerous, limited outbreaks since identification in 2003 associated with a case-fatality rate of 50%. These viruses pose an ever-present risk as they may be only a mutation away from acquiring the enhanced human-human transmission needed to be pandemic-eligible, hereby very grossly defined as pathogen with Basic Reproductive Number (R_0) > 1.

Porcine (swine) influenza viruses, such as H1N1, regularly circulate among pigs, resulting in ongoing outbreaks. Pigs may develop a mild respiratory disease upon infection, but the inflammatory response is usually limited and not associated with high mortality. Concerningly, pigs are also susceptible to infection from avian and human-borne influenza viruses. This leads to one of the greatest risks of influenza: mutation. Viruses mutate and produce variants—this has been clearly demonstrated by COVID-19. Influenza viruses are particularly prone to significant genetic mutation and alteration with risk rising substantially when animals are co-infected with several different strains. For this reason, mass animal husbandry practices such as Concentrated Animal Feeding Operations (CAFO) present a high outbreak risk by providing an ideal environment for the mixture and mutation of porcine and avian influenza viruses as well as an immediate interface for human acquisition.

Earth currently has about 8 billion inhabitants with projections estimating population growth to 9 billion by 2045. The majority of this population increase is projected occur within urban centers and has already resulted in the development of "megacities" across the globe. The United Nations defines a "megacity" as an urban center having a population in excess of 10 million. There are approximately 30–40 megacities worldwide and this number is expected to rapidly increase with most development occurring in LMIC. The inherent risk to current trends in urbanization presents an enormous public health hazard when superadded to the volatile mixture of malnutrition, fractured infrastructure, and conflict that inundate nations of the Global South. UN-Habitat estimates that approximately one-third of LMIC populations live in urban "slum" settings characterized by pathopermissive conditions of poverty, lack of sanitation, and population growth in excess of infrastructural carrying capacity. It is theorized that the Ebola virus outbreak sparked in West Africa was fanned into flame by a combination of deforestation and pathopermissive urban conditions of impoverishment. In modern day LMIC nations, as in 1848 Upper Silesia, pathopermissive urban-slum conditions introduce significant levels of biologic risk and provide fertile ground for the introduction and dissemination of contagious pathogen [53, 54, 64–68].

5.4 Outbreak's golden hour: insight from sepsis care

The theory [of sepsis] with the strongest support is that of a toxin causing [circulatory collapse via] increased capillary permeability and escape of plasma into tissue.

Dr. Walter B. Cannon, 1923. Early description of sepsis.

Sepsis is a dangerous physiologic phenomenon and one of clinical medicine's oldest and most lethal enemies. It can occur when an infection or toxin has spread from its source point into the bloodstream. The pathogen's systemic dissemination sets off a lethal cascade of events that drop blood pressure, starving the organs of oxygen. In its advanced state, sepsis leads to multisystem organ failure and death.

The importance of early action in the treatment of sepsis is paramount. Ideally, an infection is immediately treated at its point source before dissemination occurs. Once a pathogen has entered the bloodstream and initiated a septic cascade, antibiotics must be administered within 1 hour. A moribund history has taught us that after this point mortality increases significantly. These principles of medicine can theoretically be extrapolated and applied to the management of infections within our international body. As in clinical medicine, prevention of infection is the first priority. When this fails, and an infection develops, it is critical to contain the outbreak at its source before it can disseminate through our shared arteries of trade and travel. Just as in septic care, rapid, decisive, and effective action must be taken within a critical window of time to avoid bad outcomes. The "Golden Hour" of sepsis provides an example of a systems approach to ensuring critical action be taken in appropriate time. There has not been a directly analogous golden window of action that has been defined for source containment of outbreaks. The variation in pathogenicity characteristics between pathogen naturally confounds the ability to establish broad, universally applicable protocols. However, in the sections that follow, I will attempt to utilize recent modeling studies and prior zoonotic pandemic patterns to clarify a possible action window for source containment of pandemic-eligible pathogen that could be used as a starting point to help inform a standardized, systematic approach to international outbreak response [69, 70].

5.5 Insight from exercise and disease modeling

Outbreak science adapts to the emergency situation in a rapid assessment approach where evidence-making and decision-making emerge simultaneously...In the presence of uncertainty, mathematical models offer a bridge to 'knowing' by generating scenarios to enable rapid policy decisions. Projections thus afford biosecurity through calculus, by anticipating unknowns, and 'disease', into a governable present.

Rhodes et al, 2020.

Beginning with the American *Dark Winter* bioterror exercise in 2001, modeled outbreak scenarios have been undertaken regularly. It is important to note that models are artificial and unable to fully account for the complex and multifactorial nature of disease outbreaks. Mathematical models are well understood to have significant limitations and inherent uncertainty; however, they offer a unique and critical benefit in rapid pandemic response and policy making as decisions must often be made before all needed information is known. A working group of infectious disease experts and disease modeling specialists predicted that following initial index case infection, an airborne respiratory virus would be capable of spreading to infect 700,000 within the first month with complete international dissemination being possible 2 months later.

In March 2021, the Nuclear Threat Initiative and the Munich Security Conference collaborated to stage a high-level, tabletop-modeled pandemic scenario using current global infrastructure and response protocol. The scenario chosen was conservative, pre-supposing international cooperation and functional national health infrastructure. The exercise involved an unusual outbreak of monkeypox in a fictional nation with intact infrastructure. The fictional inoculation and introduction occurred during a national holiday on May 15, 2022. In June, the nation's national health department identifies and reports a novel, mutated strain of monkeypox virus to have infected 1400 citizens with four deaths reported to that date. There is no immediate evidence of international spread. An internationally supported containment response is then undertaken in an effort to establish disease source control.

The next scenario timepoint occurs 6 months later. In the interim, the international public health response had been unable to establish source control fast enough and the virus had internationally disseminated. As of January 10, 2023, the virus had spread to 83 countries with 70 million reported cases and 1.3 million fatalities. Critical trade and supply lines lay disrupted, and the global economy had come to a standstill [53, 54, 64, 71–75].

5.6 Lessons from history

> *Those who cannot remember the past are condemned to repeat it.*
>
> *George Santayana, 1863-1952.*

SARS, Ebola, and COVID-19 all-share devastating similarities and can prove historically instructive. SARS was first detected by Chinese health authorities in Guandong province on November 18, 2002. In February 2003, SARS had broken from its point of origin and was detected in Vietnam, Canada, and Hong Kong. The WHO was only officially notified of the outbreak in February with a global alert issued in March, by which time the virus had spread further to Singapore and Taiwan. In this instance, the lack of Chinese international cooperation precluded any ability to control international dissemination. The SARS coronavirus was confirmed present in more than three additional countries 4 months following initial detection.

In the case of Ebola in 2014, West African nations proved internationally cooperative but lacked the essential infrastructure necessary to achieve source control. Researchers believe that the index outbreak inoculation occurred in December 2013 in Guinea. The infection spread undetected for months until March 2014 when health officials announced an outbreak of a mysterious hemorrhagic fever virus that "strikes like lightning." That same month, Liberia reported similar cases. Medicines Sans Frontières (MSF) immediately responded but international aid was otherwise slow to follow. By April, the virus had spread to Mali followed by Sierra Leone in May. In August 2014, the disease reached the doorstep of the Global North. The United States, Spain, and the United Kingdom had active Ebolavirus cases in hospital. In the 2014

Ebola outbreak, the virus was provided an opportunity to emerge, propagate, and disseminate within a period of 4 months, largely due to pathopermissive conditions created by a resource-strapped public health system and confluent environmental risk factors. In the absence of effective national health infrastructure, source control was critically stymied, and the golden window for containment passed quickly.

COVID-19 represents the latest zoonotic pandemic. Its timeline is strikingly similar to that of SARS, but its impact has been orders of magnitude worse. COVID-19 was likely circulating in Wuhan in November of 2019. Its source of introduction remains unknown though the animal-to-human interface at wet markets and the resident institute of virology each pose known and significant infectious disease risk.

Two possible COVID-19 index cases had been identified on Nov 17 and Dec 1. The outbreak became noted by Chinese health authorities in December, but an international warning was not given. In January, China acknowledged an outbreak of acute pneumonia associated with a respiratory virus. However, conflicting reports were provided about transmissibility which proved critically misleading. By mid-January, COVID-19 had been reported in Chinese major urban centers, Thailand, Singapore, Hong Kong, Japan, France, and the United States. The WHO declared an international emergency on January 30, 2020, with the declaration of an international pandemic delayed into March. With international hands tied by disinformation and lack of cooperation, COVID-19 was able to rapidly disseminate from its point of origin and become internationally systemic within a period of 3 months.

An examination of modeling scenarios and pandemic trends in aggregate reveal a disturbingly common theme: We are consistently too late. By the time international support has been mustered and action has been taken, the horses are well out of the barn. SARS, Ebola, COVID-19, and pathogen modeling studies demonstrate a consistent ability for pandemic-eligible pathogen to internationally disseminate within approximately 3 months if source control is not achieved. This gross, roughly estimated 2–3 month "Golden Window" of outbreak response may be decisive in determining whether or not a pandemic-eligible pathogen will be able to be contained within its region of introduction. The above-proposed window is only a rough sketch generated from relatively scant data. Further, rigorous clarification of a pandemic response timeline may prove very beneficial in systematically orienting and organizing decisive and timely international response to outbreak containment [53, 54, 76–78].

5.7 One health, one risk, one future

It is the microbes that have the last word.

Louis Pasteur.

Due to our shared elements of vulnerability, there is an urgent need for international cooperative endeavors to promote and preserve health since [Emerging Infectious Disease] no know geographic or economic borders.

M. J. Tosam et al. 2019

Humanity stands at an ethical and existential crossroads and time is of the essence. Every minute a Somali child is admitted for severe malnutrition. The next, another has perished from malaria. At the end of the day, at least 800 more have been lost to preventable, diarrheal illness.

The development and integrity of LMIC nations of the Global South are actively being undermined by preventable disease, intrastate conflict, and climatic catastrophe. Our shared world continues to be repeatedly challenged by preventable pandemics that are proving increasingly devastating over time. COVID-19, the latest pandemic iteration, has not been controlled and is now moving toward global endemicity. All the while, the risk of another internationally paralytic pandemic from EID remains at a historic high and the stumbling blocks that stymied our prior containment responses to SARS, Ebola, and COVID remain present.

We live in an era of unprecedented risk that is shared by all members of our international body. The crises jeopardizing our global health security are interrelated and complex, but the solutions that have been defined are relatively elegant in principle: We must expediently invest in the empowering, sustainable development of our neighbors in the Global South. The health security of our international body will require all member nations to be developmentally healed and infrastructurally functional. Central organ systems critical to global homeostasis must also be operational and properly funded. It will be only through solidarity that we can hope to effectively and sustainably safeguard the health of our international community [9, 53, 54, 79].

Acknowledgements

I am a new author and a trainee in the field of preventive medicine and public health. In helping to usher this call to action, I stand on the shoulders of giants in the field who have clarified the present threats and defined potential solutions. This chapter was able to be completed only with the support of a village of mentors and colleagues. I would first like to sincerely thank IntechOpen for their dedication to Open Access publishing and information equity; and for the privilege and opportunity to contribute to a discussion and topic that is my passion. I would also like to thank the faculty of the University of California San Diego (UCSD) Preventive Medicine Residency Program and San Diego State University (SDSU) School of Public Health (SPH) for the phenomenal education I have been provided and for the faculty support I've received throughout this process. I'd like especially to thank SDSU SPH Divisions of Epidemiology & Biostatistics and Environmental Health for providing me invaluable preparation for the writing of this chapter.

I deeply thank my colleagues who have critically aided me in writing, including but certainly not limited to: Chief Editor Mr. Isaiah Briggs of Harvard Divinity School, Lead Editors: Mr. Joshua Kapusinski author of The Awakening (2022), and Ms. Maria Alexandra Hernandez and Mr. Haider Ghiasuddin of Geisel School of Medicine at Dartmouth for their invaluable assistance.

I would like to thank Mr. Antonio Guterres and Mr. Volodymyr Zelenskyy for their outstanding and truly inspirational international and national leadership during this time of extraordinary crisis. I would also like to thank MIT Emeritus Professor of Linguistics Noam Chomsky, as well as the late Yale Professor of Law, Arthur Allen Leff (1935–1981), for the pivotal role they have played in my (and many others) intellectual and academic development. I thank Al Jazeera for their excellent and equitable coverage of global news, and for making a point to uplift the voices of those seldom heard. I deeply admire and thank Medicines Sans Frontiers (MSF) for their critical and relentless work aiding migrants and refugees, and for MSF's consistent, strong advocacy for the world's underserved. Finally, I would like to thank and acknowledge Mr. Nikola Tesla (1856–1943) for his inspiringly genuine and wonderful approach to nature and science, and most importantly, for his revolutionary development of the Alternating Current that powers our world and for which he is seldom recognized.

This chapter is written for, and dedicated to, my brothers and sisters in the Global South, who have endured unfathomable, preventable suffering for centuries without reason. I am an incredibly insufficient author in advocating for the prompt and sustainable development of LMIC; however, I do hope that this chapter can direct attention and action toward this goal as it is critical to the preservation of global health security. I pray the human species will find the moral courage required to heal our neighbors and ensure a safe tomorrow for our children. This chapter represents an independent work generously supported through the IntechOpen expanded sponsorship opportunity program.

Conflict of interest

The author declares no conflict of interest.

Notes/thanks/other declarations

In closing, I would like to thank my Mom and Dad, who have worked hard to provide my little brother and I with opportunities that were not available for them.

Author details

Aaron Briggs
PGY2 UCSD Preventive Medicine Residency Program, University of California San Diego, San Diego, CA, USA

*Address all correspondence to: ambriggs@health.ucsd.edu

References

[1] IMF Communications Department. Annual Meetings Update. Washington: International Monetary Fund; 14 Oct 2022. Available from: https://www.imf.org/en/News/Seminars/Campaigns/2022/10/Annual-Meetings-Day5-2

[2] Guterres A. United Nations Common Agenda Report. UN Secretariat. New York, USA; 2022

[3] Walsh PP, Banerjee A, Murphy E. The UN 2030 agenda for sustainable development. In: Partnerships and the Sustainable Development Goals. Cham: Springer; 2022. pp. 1-12

[4] Mecklin J. Science and Security Board Bulletin of the Atomic Scientists. At doom's Doorstep: It Is 100 Seconds to Midnight: 2022 Doomsday Clock Statement. Oxfordshire, England: Francis & Taylor Publishing; 20 Jan 2022

[5] Rawls J. A theory of justice. In: Ethics. Oxfordshire, England, UK: Routledge; 2004. pp. 229-234

[6] Darwin C. The Voyage of the Beagle. London, New York, Dent; Dutton; 1959. pp. 1809-1882

[7] Timaeus of Tauromenium (356-260BC). The Lost History of Sicily: 'The Sword of Damocles.' Greece

[8] Guterres A. United Nations General Assembly 77th Session. UN Secretariat. New York, USA: Opening Press Conference; 2022

[9] Chowdhury Z. San Diego State University: Public Health Course 604: Environmental Determinants of Health. Infectious Disease and Environmental Determinants of Health Lecture Series. San Diego, CA; 2021

[10] Assembly UG. Universal declaration of human rights. UN General Assembly. 1948;**302**(2):14-25

[11] South Sudanese Woman. Interview re: African Drought & Climate Change. Doha, Qatar: Al Jazeera; 2022

[12] Ghebreyesus T. Vaccine Inequity Undermining Global Economic Recovery. Geneva/New York City: WHO/UN Joint News Release; 2021

[13] IPCC. Climate Change 2021: The Physical Science Basis. Contribution of Working Group I to the Sixth Assessment Report of the Intergovernmental Panel on Climate Change. In: Masson-Delmotte V, Zhai P, Pirani A, Connors SL, Péan C, Berger S, et al, editors. Cambridge, United Kingdom: Cambridge University Press and New York, NY, USA; 2021. DOI: 10.1017/9781009157896 [In press]

[14] World Health Organization. Global Conference on Health and Climate Change. Geneva, Switzerland: WHO Press; 2021

[15] Chancel L, Piketty T, Saez E. World Inequality Report. Cambridge, USA: Harvard University Press; 2022

[16] Fanon F, Sartre JP, Farrington C. The Wretched of the Earth. Vol. 36. New York: Grove Press; 1963

[17] UN General Assembly 77th Session. UN Secretariat. New York, USA: Secretary General Guterres Opening Press Release; 2022

[18] Hesoid. Prometheus. 600-700 BC. Greece

[19] Beall EF. Hesiod's Prometheus and development in myth. Journal of the History of Ideas. 1991;**52**(3):355-371

[20] Woman K. Interview re: African Drought & Climate Change. Doha, Qatar: Al Jazeera; 2022

[21] World Food Programme. A Global Food Crisis. WFP. 2022. Available from: https://www.wfp.org/global-hunger-crisis

[22] World Health Organization. United Nations Children's Fund. Half of Health Care Facilities Globally Lack Basic Hygiene Services. Joint News Release. Geneva, Switzerland: WHO Press; 2022

[23] World Health Organization. United Nations Children's Fund. 1 in 3 People Globally Do Not Have Access to Safe Drinking Water. Joint News Release. Geneva, Switzerland: WHO Press; 2019

[24] Gallup JL, Sachs JD. The Economic Burden of Malaria. The Intolerable Burden of Malaria: A New Look at the Numbers. American Society of Tropical Medicine and Hygeine. Northbrook, IL. CID Working Paper Series; 2001;**64**

[25] Woman I. Interview re: 130 Indonesian Children Dead from Acute Kidney Failure. Doha, Qatar: Al Jazeera; 2022

[26] Oleribe OO, Momoh J, Uzochukwu BS, Mbofana F, Adebiyi A, Barbera T, et al. Identifying key challenges facing healthcare systems in Africa and potential solutions. International Journal of General Medicine. 2019;**12**:395

[27] Kruk ME, Gage AD, Arsenault C, Jordan K, Leslie HH, Roder-DeWan S, et al. High-quality health systems in the sustainable development goals era: Time for a revolution. The Lancet Global Health. 2018;**6**(11):e1196-e1252

[28] Mills A. Health care systems in low-and middle-income countries. New England Journal of Medicine. 2014;**370**(6):552-557

[29] Summit NM. Millennium Development Goals. Human Development Report; 2000

[30] The World Bank Group Partnership Fund for the Sustainable Development Goals Annual Report 2019. New York, USA: SDG Fund

[31] Review of Climate Catastrophe in Pakistan. UNICEF Report Featured. Doha, Qatar: Al Jazeera; 2022

[32] Pakistani man ('flood victim'). Interview re: Flooding & Catastrophe in Pakistan. Doha, Qatar: Al Jazeera; 2022

[33] Cederman LE, Pengl Y. Global Conflict Trends and their Consequences. United Nations: Department of Economics and Social Affairs working paper; 2019. Available from: https://www.un.org/development/desa/dpad/wpcontent/uploads/sites/45/publication/SDO_BP_Cederman_Pengl.pdf

[34] Bell E, Cullen J, Taylor S. United Nations/Framework Convention on Climate Change. Adoption of the Paris agreement, 21st Conference of the Parties, Paris: United Nations. An Official Publication; 2015

[35] Leonard M, Blackhurst R. I don't think anybody thought much about whether Agent Orange was against the rules of war. The Observer. Kings Place, London. 19 May 2002

[36] Lloyd Marion. Soviets Close to Using A-Bomb in 1962 Crisis, Forum is Told. The Boston Globe. 13 Oct 2002

[37] Chomsky N. Hegemony or Survival: America's Quest for Global Dominance. New York, NY: Henry Holt and Company; 2003

[38] UN News. UN chief calls for an end to 'nuclear blackmail' and risk

of 'humanitarian Armageddon'. UN Secretariat. New York, USA; 26 Sep 2022

[39] Al Jazeera News Agency. Russia to Send Belarus Nuclear-Capable Missiles within Months. Doha, Qatar: Aljazeera, Russia-Ukraine War News Release; 25 Jun 2022

[40] Woolf AF. The New START Treaty: Central Limits and Key Provisions. Library of Congress Congressional Research Service. Washington, D.C.; 2014

[41] Goldblat J. The biological weapons convention: An overview. International Review of the Red Cross (1961-1997). 1997;**37**(318):251-265

[42] Convention on the Prohibition of the Development, Production, Stockpiling and Use of Chemical Weapons and on their Destruction. 13 Jan 1993. 1974 UNTS 45; 32 ILM 800

[43] Rietiker D, Mohr M, Yamada T. Treaty on the prohibition of nuclear weapons. A short commentary article by article. In: International Association of Lawyers against Nuclear Arms (IALANA). Berlin, Germany; 2018. pp. 10-11

[44] UN News. Chief Disappointed Nuclear Treaty Conference Ends without Consensus. New York, USA: Peace and Security Press Release; 27 Aug 2022

[45] Guterres A. UN General Assembly 77th Session. UN Secretariat. New York, USA: Security Council High-Level Meeting on the Sahel; 2022

[46] UN News. Black Sea Grain Exports Deal 'a Beacon of Hope' amid Ukraine War. New York, USA: Peace and Security Press Release; 22 July 2022

[47] Guterres A. UN General Assembly 77th Session. New York, USA: UN Secretariat, Security Council High-Level Meeting on the Sahel; 2022

[48] Sudanese Minister of Social Welfare. Interview re: Blue Nile State Violence. Doha, Qatar: Al Jazeera; 2022

[49] Caseloads R. World Economic Outlook. World Economic Outlook; 2022

[50] Elnagar R, Calvino N. Annual meetings of the IMF and the World Bank. In: Concluding Remarks. IMF Communications Department. Washington DC, USA. 2022

[51] Virchow RC. Archiv für pathologische Anatomie und Physiologie und für klinische Medicin. Vol. 2. Berlin, Germany: George Reimer; 1848. pp. 143-332

[52] Virchow RC. Report on the typhus epidemic in upper Silesia. American Journal of Public Health. 2006;**96**(12):2102-2105

[53] Quick JD, Fryer B. The End of Epidemics: The Looming Threat to Humanity and How to Stop it. New York, NY: St. Martin's Press; 2018

[54] Gostin LO. Global Health Security: A Blueprint for the Future. Cambridge, MA: Harvard University Press; 2021

[55] Hansen C, Paintsil E. Infectious diseases of poverty in children: A tale of two worlds. Pediatric Clinics. 2016;**63**(1):37-66

[56] In Danger: UNAIDS Global AIDS Update 2022. Geneva: Joint United Nations Programme on HIV/ AIDS; 2022. Licence: CC BY-NC-SA 3.0 IGO

[57] WHO Global Tuberculosis Report 2022. Global tuberculosis report. Geneva, Switzerland: WHO Press; 2022

[58] WHO Malaria Overview. 2022. Available from: https://www.who.int/news-room/fact-sheets/detail/malaria [Accessed: October 2022]

[59] Arrow KJ, Panosian C, Gelband H. The human and economic burden of malaria. In: Saving Lives, Buying Time: Economics of Malaria Drugs in an Age of Resistance. Washington, D.C.: National Academies Press (US); 2004

[60] Shang W, Wang Y, Yuan J, Guo Z, Liu J, Liu M. Global excess mortality during COVID-19 pandemic: A systematic review and meta-analysis. Vaccines. 2022;**10**(10):1702

[61] Laiton-Donato K, Usme-Ciro JA, Franco-Muñoz C, Álvarez-Díaz DA, Ruiz-Moreno HA, Reales-González J, et al. Novel highly divergent SARS-CoV-2 lineage with the spike substitutions L249S and E484K. Frontiers in Medicine. 2021;**8**:932

[62] Lorenzo-Redondo R, Ozer EA, Hultquist JF. Covid-19: Is omicron less lethal than delta? BMJ. 2022;**378**

[63] Kominers S, et al. It's time to redouble and refocus our efforts to fight covid, not retreat. BMJ. 2022;**379**:o2423. DOI: 10.1136/bmj.o2423

[64] Pakistani man (flood victim). Interview re: Catastrophe & Spreading Disease in Pakistan. Doha, Qatar: Al Jazeera; 2022

[65] Yassif J, Isaac C, & O'Prey KP. Strengthening global systems to prevent and respond to high-consequence biological threats. NTI report. 2021. Available from: https://www.nti.org/wp-content/uploads/2021/11/NTI_Paper_BIO-TTX_Final.pdf

[66] Tosam MJ, Ambe JR, Chi PC. Global emerging pathogens, poverty and vulnerability: An ethical analysis. Socio-cultural Dimensions of Emerging Infectious Diseases in Africa. An indigenous response to deadly epidemics. 2019:243-253. DOI: 10.1007/978-3-030-17474-3_18

[67] United States Center for Disease Control: Avian Flu. Webpage Page last reviewed. 2022. Available from: https://www.cdc.gov/flu/avianflu/index.htm [Accessed: October 2022]

[68] United States Center for Disease Control: Information on Swine/Variant Influenza. Webpage Page last reviewed. 2022. Available from: https://www.cdc.gov/flu/avianflu/index.htm [Accessed: October 2022]

[69] Burchard KW. The Clinical Handbook for Surgical Critical Care. Boca Raton, FL: CRC Press; 2012

[70] Garg SK. Hit hard in golden hours: Thoughts on preventing the next pandemic. New Microbes and New Infections. 2022;**48**

[71] Rhodes T, Lancaster K, Lees S, Parker M. Modelling the pandemic: Attuning models to their contexts. BMJ Global Health. 2020;**5**(6):e002914

[72] O'Toole T, Mair M, Inglesby TV. Shining light on "Dark Winter". Clinical Infectious Diseases. 2002;**34**:972-983

[73] Smith BT, Inglesby TV, Brimmer E, Borio L, Franco C, Gronvall GK, et al. Navigating the storm: Report and recommendations from the Atlantic storm exercise. Biosecurity and Bioterrorism: Biodefense Strategy, Practice, and Science. 2005;**3**(3):256-267

[74] Hellewell J, Abbott S, Gimma A, Bosse NI, Jarvis CI, Russell TW, et al. Feasibility of controlling COVID-19 outbreaks by isolation of cases and contacts. The Lancet Global Health. 2020;**8**(4):e488-e496

[75] Kamorudeen RT, Adedokun KA, Olarinmoye AO. Ebola outbreak in West Africa, 2014-2016: Epidemic timeline, differential diagnoses, determining

factors, and lessons for future response. Journal of Infection and Public Health. 2020;**13**(7):956-962

[76] Santayana G. The Life of Reason: Reason in Society. Vol. 2. New York, NY: C. Scribner's Sons; 1905

[77] Frost M, Li R, Moolenaar R, Mao QA, Xie R. Progress in public health risk communication in China: Lessons learned from SARS to H7N9. BMC Public Health. 2019;**19**(3):1-9

[78] World Health Organization, editor. 83 SARS: Lessons from a new disease. In: Shaping the Future. Geneva, Switzerland: WHO Press – World Health Organization; 2003. pp. 71-82

[79] Tosam MJ, Ambe JR, Chi PC. Global emerging pathogens, poverty and vulnerability: An ethical analysis. In: Socio-Cultural Dimensions of Emerging Infectious Diseases in Africa. Cham: Springer; 2019. pp. 243-253

Section 2

Access to Health Services for Important Health Problems

Chapter 3

Funding of Oncology Benefits by Medical Schemes, South Africa: A Focus on Breast and Cervical Cancer

Michael Mncedisi Willie, Thulisile Noutchang, Maninie Molatseli and Sipho Kabane

Abstract

Breast and cervical cancers are among the top five worldwide. The mortality rate for breast cancer is over 50%, when compared to cervical cancer, which is nearly 90%. Early breast and cervical cancer screening can reduce mortality risk. This study examined breast and cervical cancer rates among South African medical scheme members. The study's secondary goal was to analyse how medical schemes funded these two cancers, including patient and/or out-of-pocket payments, to identify funding gaps. The study was a cross-sectional retrospective review of medical scheme claims data for oncology benefits, especially for breast and cervical cancers. The study used a multivariate logistic regression model to assess cancer rates. The results showed that the relative proportion of beneficiaries with breast cancer was higher in open schemes than restricted, in large schemes than medium and small schemes, in comprehensive plans, efficiency discount options (EDOs), hospital plans than in partial cover plans, in age groups older than 55, in an out-of-hospital setting than in in-hospital setting. The paper advises examining the funding mechanism of oncology benefits to reduce out-of-pocket payments (OOPs) for cancer patients, revising network arrangements, and using designated service provider (DSP) as a barrier to access against uneven oncology provider distribution.

Keywords: breast cancer, cervical cancer, prescribed minimum benefits, diagnostic treatment pairs benefits paid, mental healthcare access

1. Introduction

Cervical and breast cancers threaten the lives of many women, accounting for two million newly diagnosed cases and 800,000 cancer-related deaths annually [1]. The incidence rate of cervical and breast cancer is much greater in low- and middle-income countries (LMICs) than in industrialised nations, where screening facilities and other preventive treatments are readily available [2–6]. Compared to low-income countries, high-income countries have significantly raised screening rates [7, 8]. In the World Health Organization Regional Office for Africa WHO (AFRO) African area, screening rates are still relatively low [7, 8]. In addition, 90% of cervical cancer deaths occur in women residing in low- and middle-income countries (LMICs), with sub-Saharan Africa bearing the heaviest burden [6, 9]. In South Africa, cervical and breast screening uptake disparities are caused by a lack of education and access to information. A study in Korea also showed that breast and cervical cancer screening rates varied widely among women with higher household incomes and education levels [1]. Other variables, such as limited access to health care facilities, lack of knowledge and health promotion, and inadequate support and awareness programmes for women, which are more prevalent in less affluent rural areas, influence early detection, diagnosis, and screening uptake [10, 11]. Recent research has shown that metropolitan location remains a significant factor related to greater awareness of cervical cancer risk factors, resulting in lower screening rates in rural regions [11–13]. In addition, lack of access to facilities in rural locations adds to inadequate screening services, a barrier to an admission that results in delayed seeking behaviour. Studies have demonstrated that early screening helps in detecting cervical cancer early [14]. The availability and accessibility of early screening and treatment services contribute to the notable disparities in cervical and breast cancer incidence. Early detection through screening and surveillance should be linked to available resources for treatment, such as access to providers and facilities [15, 16]. The author further warns that careful consideration must be paid to ensure that all aspects of cancer control programmes are balanced to limit unintended harm [15].

Other factors linked to health systems are human resources challenges, the scarcity of specialist services, and the uneven distribution of specialists by sector. Studies have shown that most specialists for oncology-related services are concentrated in the private sector rather than in the public sector [17]. In South Africa, nearly 80% of oncology specialists (radiation oncologists) practice in the private sector, are mainly remunerated through the funding model of medical schemes (health insurance providers), and cater for 16% of the population [18, 19]. The remaining 20% of the specialists cater to 84% of the population. **Figure 1** further illustrates inequities in the distribution of oncology service providers and how they have evolved over the last 3 years, showing a consistent trend toward an increasing share in the private sector.

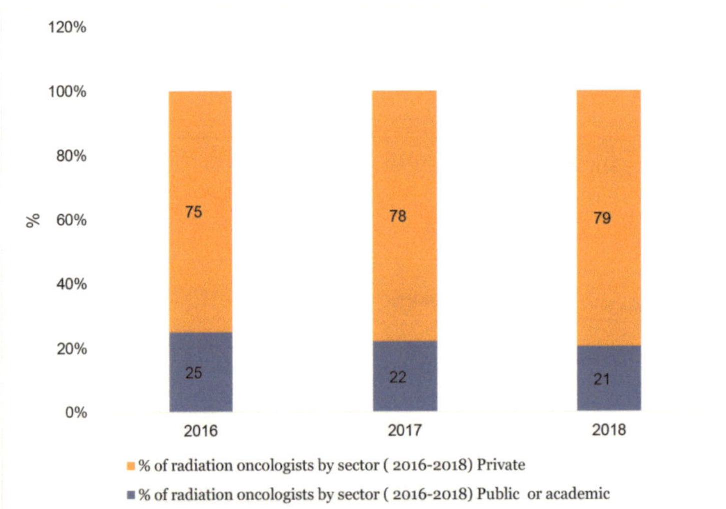

Figure 1.
Distribution of radiation oncologists by sector-South Africa. Source: Adapted from Abratt [17].

2. Breast cancer

Breast cancer is the most common cancer among women and the top cause of death in more than 100 countries worldwide [20–22]. Over 2 million new breast cancer cases have been detected worldwide, representing a quarter of all cancer cases in women [20, 23, 24]. The incidence of breast cancer in the WHO's African region (AFRO) accounts for 27.7 percent of all cancer cases, and there are 29,593 breast cancer patients in South Africa [20, 22, 25]. The high incidence rates in affluent and developing nations are driven by non-genetic risk factors associated with menstruation, reproduction, exogenous hormone replacement, alcohol consumption, and weight gain [20, 26–28]. Age and gender are risk factors associated with breast cancer; the incidence of breast cancer increases and is more prevalent in women aged 50 or older than in men. Madeira et al. [29] stated that men account for 1% of all breast cancer cases [30, 31]. The average age of a breast cancer diagnosis varies according to gender. In a systematic analysis of 1,201 male breast cancer patients from 27 African nations, Ndom et al. [32] showed that the average age for men was 54.6 years, and for women, it was 47.7 years. Baudouin Kongolo Kakudji et al. [33] created an epidemiological, clinical, and diagnostic profile of breast cancer patients treated at the regional hospital in Potchefstroom, South Africa. The study's majority of patients (98.6 percent) were female, with a mean age of 56.2 years (standard deviation: 14.4) (95 percent confidence interval: (54.6–59.7) [33]. The average cost of breast cancer therapy varies by location or geographic area; sector, setting (in and out of hospital), treatment modality and level of care, disease severity, and disease stage [34]. The expected cost of chemotherapy in the South African public sector is R15,740 [34]. The average cost of medical treatment for breast cancer in each episode in South Africa is imprecise, and the available data contain methodological flaws. Finestone et al. [27] demonstrate that the average cost of breast cancer in the private sector was more than three times that of the public sector. During the first year after a breast cancer diagnosis, Discovery Health Medical Scheme (DHMS) estimated the average cost to treat breast cancer to be in the region of R207 561 [35]. Finestone et al. [27] estimate that the cost varies with stage, with the estimated cost for stage 1 in the private sector being R352 495 and the

Diagnosis	Treatment
• Mammogram - R1 800 • Ultrasound - R1 400 • MRI scans and CT scans - R3 000 – R15 000 • Stereotactic biopsy - R4 000 to R6 000 • Oncotype DX (one type of genetic testing) - R30 000	Surgical • Lumpectomy - R30 000 • Mastectomy of both breasts with reconstruction - R150 000 – R250 000. Non-surgical • Hormone treatments such as Tamoxifen can be reasonable at R100 a month. • A drug such as Herceptin can cost around R20 000 for one dose, which can be prescribed monthly. • A session of radiation therapy and/or chemotherapy could cost from a few thousand to over R10 000

Source: Adapted from 1Life [36]: data excludes additional and aftercare: ongoing follow-up doctors' visits and health checks and tests

Table 1.
Estimated cost of medical treatment of breast cancer (Diagnosis and Treatment).

projected cost for stage 4 being significantly higher at R522 553. Indicating a variation between health plans or benefit options, the author confirmed that the cost was considerably lower for low-cost benefit alternatives [27]. The costs vary based on diagnosis and therapy, as shown in **Table 1**.

3. Cervical cancer

In 2020, cervical cancer was the fourth most prevalent cancer in women worldwide, with a projected incidence of more than 600,000 cases and over 350,000 deaths [21, 22]. Cervical cancer incidence and mortality rates are the greatest in Africa, notably in Southern, Eastern, and Western Africa [25]. Cervical cancer is the most common in many sub-Saharan African countries (22 percent of all cancers), and its prevalence in poor developing countries is potentially 15 times higher. After breast cancer, cervical cancer accounts for 18.7 percent of all cancer incidences in South Africa's female population [22, 27]. The incidence of cervical cancer increases with age, with the average age of diagnosis ranging from 35 to 44. The average age of cervical cancer diagnosis in South Africa is 45 [37]. Due to the greater prevalence of cervical cancer in women with HIV, which is more prevalent in younger women, it is suggested that younger women get cervical cancer screening at an early age. Cervical cancer is diagnosed at an average age of 50 to 53 years [38]. A study conducted in South Africa revealed a significantly lower average age of 40.8 years (SD 18.6, range 15–95 years); nevertheless, the analysis concentrated on 5,903 females (15–49 years) [39]. Similarly to breast cancer, the average cost of medical therapy for cervical cancer varies by sector, setting (in and out of hospital), treatment modality, level of care, disease severity, and disease stage [37, 39]. In the private sector, the average cost of cervical cancer was 9 times greater for stage 1 and 13 times greater for stage 4 [27]. The limitations of the study by Finestone et al. [27] were that it contrasted one medical scheme to the public sector, excluding closed schemes like the Government Employees Medical Scheme (GEMS), which primarily serves public sector personnel; other medical schemes were also excluded in the analysis. Similarly, non-included plans may have a specific risk and age profile.

4. Legislative requirements

The level of care for breast and cervical (oncology) services (**Table 2**) is outlined in the Council of Medical Schemes Act's Prescribed Minimum Benefit (PMB) list [40]. PMBs are defined benefits designed to ensure that all members of medical plans have access to some fundamental health care, regardless of the benefit option selected. The PMB list consists of 25 Chronic Disease List (CDL) diseases and an additional 271 Diagnosis and Treatment Pair (DTP) conditions. Regarding breast and cervical cancer services, medical schemes must cover the diagnosis, treatment, and care for these disorders. However, medical schemes are not required to pay for diagnostic tests to determine that a patient does not have a PMB illness. Cervical cancer screening is a PMB level of service under DTP Code 960M. The treatment component of breast cancer screening includes PMB-level periodic breast examinations. However, members are entitled to specific screening intervals, instruments, and HPV versus cervical screening. **Table 2** demonstrates the optimal amount of care recommended by the regulator [40].

	Cervical cancer	Breast cancer
Screening	Pap smears	Mammography
Diagnosis	1. Consultations with GPs (1) and specialists (4) for a diagnosis, staging and risk assessment of cancer. 2. Radiology 3. Pathology (Full blood count, liver/renal function, Creatinine, HIV)	1. Consultations with a nurse or GP (1) and specialists (4) for a cancer diagnosis, staging and risk assessments. 2. Radiology (mammogram, ultrasound) 3. Pathology (Full blood count, liver/renal function)
Staging	1. Additional pathology where necessary 2. Imaging radiology (ultrasound, X-ray, CT, MRI*, PET*)	1. Imaging radiology (chest X-ray, liver ultrasound, CT, MRI)
Treatment	Stage 1: Biopsy, Hysterectomy Stage 2: Hysterectomy, lymphadenectomy Stage 3: Chemoradiotherapy, chemoradiation Stage 4: Radiotherapy	Breast-conserving surgery Systemic therapy Radiotherapy Management of advanced disease (hormone therapy, chemotherapy)

Source: CMS [40]

Table 2.
Level of care for breast and cervical (oncology) services.

5. Funding models (benefit design)

Most oncology treatments are provided in-hospital and subject to network hospitals and designated service providers (DSPs), with some entry-level plans using the state as a DSP. Entry-level coverage plans typically cover oncology care at the PMB level. Oncology coverage includes PMBs in their entirety. Schemes provide different cancer treatment limits and extended benefits for more complete benefit options. However, after the annual maximum is reached, patients may be required to pay co-payments for treatment exceeding PMB level care (which costs more than the scheme rate). The oncology benefit does not cover hospital admissions; these are paid by the hospital benefit of the benefit choice the patient is enrolled in. After this hospital benefit has been exhausted, patients may be required to continue treatment at an entry-level network institution or a state facility. Most medical schemes include cancer benefits, annual limits for oncology treatment, and entry-level benefit alternatives for PMB-level care. Comparatively, comprehensive plans cover R400,000 or more [41–43]. ICON Oncology is the major designated service provider with regard to out-of-hospital benefits [19]. Nonetheless, in-hospital benefits are accessible through the state as a DSP (for some entry-level alternatives) and private institutions (subject to annual hospital limits).

6. Objectives

This study's primary purpose was to investigate the rates of breast and cervical cancer among South African medical scheme beneficiaries. The secondary purpose of the study was to analyse the funding model of these two types of diagnoses by medical schemes, including measuring the level of pocket payments made by these patients to identify funding gaps, and lastly, to execute a logistic regression model to identify the factors that contribute to the greater exposure rates of the two types of cancer.

7. Methods

The study design was a retrospective cross-sectional investigation of medical schemes' claims data associated with oncology benefits, primarily breast and cervical cancer. The review period was 2019, and the secondary data came from the annual submissions of aggregated CMS statutory returns data. During the evaluation period, the analysis comprised claims data from 59 medical schemes with comprehensive expenditure data. There were 15 open schemes and 44 closed schemes. Breast cancer and cervical cancer were represented in the study by 47 886 and 4 116 participants,

	Description
Dependent Variable (DV)	**Rate of breast and cervical cancer.** The rate was higher than a specified cut-off points for each type of cancer: Cancer of the Cervix (0.45 per 1000) beneficiaries and cancer of the breast (2.74 per 1000).
Independent Variables (INDV)	Demographic characteristics Age bands
	A medical scheme is a non-profit organisation with a board of trustees that must be registered with the Council for Medical Schemes. In exchange for a monthly contribution or premium, medical schemes in South Africa provide members with coverage for their medical expenses. **Scheme Type:** (Open Schemes, Restricted Schemes). The Medical Schemes Act of 1998 defines open schemes as open membership. As a result, they accept anyone who wants to become a member and pay the premium (Medical Schemes Act 131 of 1998). Closed or restricted medical schemes are limited to an employer or union (Medical Schemes Act 131 of 1998).
	Scheme Size: A large scheme has more than 30,000 beneficiaries. A medium scheme has less than 30,000 beneficiaries and more than more than 6,000. A small scheme has fewer than 6,000 members [44].
	Geographic distribution of beneficiaries in the nine provinces in South Africa: Gauteng, Western Cape, KwaZulu Natal, Eastern Cape, Northern Cape, Limpopo, Free State, North West.
	Benefit design: Benefits options (Health plans) were reclassified into the following categories to assess the effect of benefits option richness [45]. • Comprehensive Plans: Provide comprehensive cover for almost all medical costs, including unlimited hospital cover and generous benefits for day-to-day expenses. • EDOs: Efficiency Discounted Options (or "EDOs") offer an appealing value proposition to medical scheme members. • Hospital Plans: Supplementary in-hospital benefits relative to PMB; no out-of-hospital (OOH) benefits • Partial Cover Plans: Partial cover for OOH benefits from risk, savings account, and no above-threshold benefits (ATB).
	Setting: In- and out-of-hospital benefits
Benefits paid/ expenditure	Expenditure reported in South African Currency: 1$= ZAR17
Out-of-pocket (OOP)	The proxy measures are determined as the difference between what the medical service provider claimed and what the medical scheme paid. Out-of-pocket is the maximum amount that you could pay for covered medical expenses in a year. This amount includes deductibles, copays (co-payments), and coinsurance.

Table 3.
Description of variables of interest.

respectively. 97% more women than men had breast cancer. Based on study and calculation, 46,571 female beneficiaries older than 20 were diagnosed with breast cancer. We counted and proportioned categorical variables. Unadjusted comparisons were statistically significant at p value <0.05. The study used a multivariate logistic regression model to examine cancer risk variables. **Table 3** shows model dependent and independent variables. The analyses were done in STATA and SAS 9.4.

8. Results

The average age of female beneficiaries with breast cancer was 59 years, whereas the age profile of female industry beneficiaries was substantially younger at 34 years. The breast cancer rate was, therefore, 14 per 1000 female beneficiaries. In the age range of 20 to 24 years, the rates were fewer than 1 per 1000 female beneficiaries, which was significantly lower than those for older age groups. In age groups 65–69, 70–74, 75–79, and 80–84, the breast cancer incidence rate was greater than 30 per 1000 female beneficiaries (**Figure 2**).

In addition, the analysed schemes accounted for 4,103 female beneficiaries diagnosed with cervical cancer who were 20 or older. Thus, the rate of breast cancer was 1.25 per 1,000 female beneficiaries. The average age of female beneficiaries diagnosed with breast cancer was 50 years, whereas the age profile of female industry beneficiaries was substantially younger at 34 years. Less than one per thousand female beneficiaries were between 20 and 24 years of age. The cervical's cancer rate was significantly greater in women aged 45 to 49, exceeding 3.3% per 1000 female beneficiaries (**Figure 3**).

Figure 4 shows the distribution of beneficiaries diagnosed with breast cancer and cancer of the cervix. The analysis shows that there were more beneficiaries with breast cancer than cervical cancer in Gauteng (41% vs 33%) and Western Cape (21% vs 9%). There were more beneficiaries with cancer of the cervix than those with cancer of the breast, 17% and 12%, respectively. However, in other provinces, such as KwaZulu Natal, a more notable difference was in Limpopo province (13% vs 5%) and Mpumalanga (8% vs 4%) (**Table 4**).

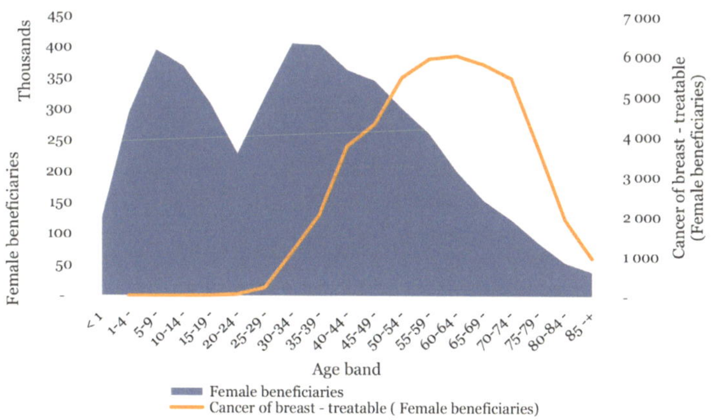

Figure 2.
Number of female beneficiaries vs cancer of breast – treatable beneficiaries.

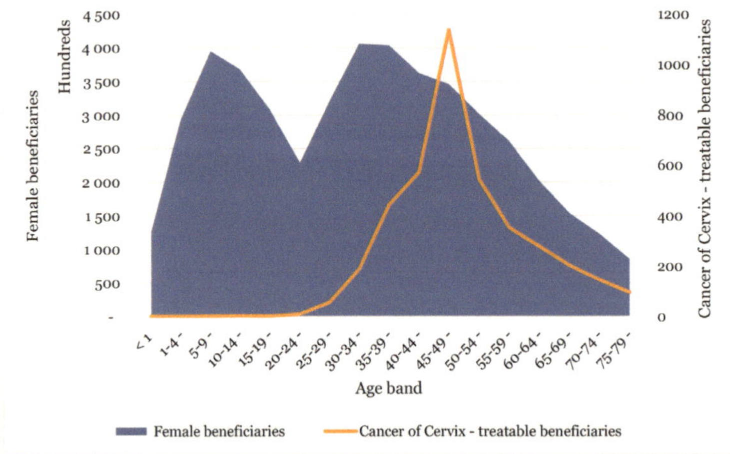

Figure 3.
Number of female beneficiaries vs cancer of breast – treatable beneficiaries.

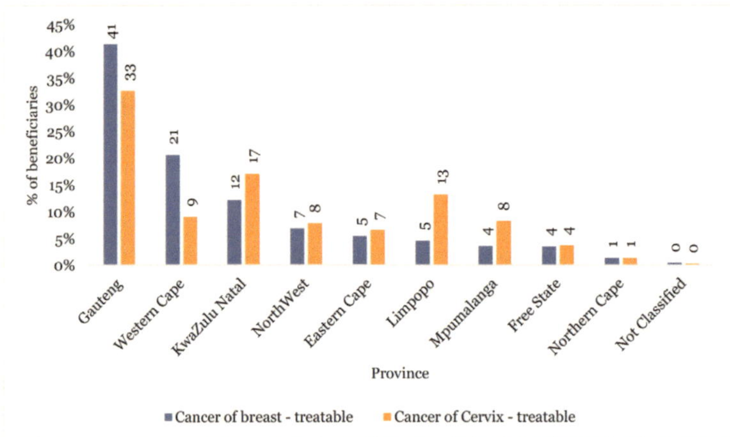

Figure 4.
Distribution of beneficiaries diagnosed with breast cancer and cancer of the cervix.

	Cancer of the breast (N = 47,886) n (%)	Cancer of the cervix (N = 4,116) n (%)	% Difference
Scheme type			
Open	30 111 (62.88)	1 698 (53.55)	−17%
Restricted	17 775 (37.11)	2 418 (46.44)	20%
Scheme size			
Large	44 912 (93.78)	3 919 (89.86)	−4%
Medium	1 978 (4.13)	130 (6.29)	34%
Small	996 (2.07)	67 (3.84)	46%
Benefit design strata			-
Comprehensive Plans	20 913 (43.67)	1 613 (39.18)	−11%

	Cancer of the breast (N = 47,886) n (%)	Cancer of the cervix (N = 4,116) n (%)	% Difference
EDOs	3 588 (7.49)	268 (6.511)	−15%
Hospital Plans	11 199 (23.38)	648 (15.74)	−49%
Partial Cover Plans	10 906 (22.77)	1 482 (36.00)	37%
Unknowns/ Not classified	1 280 (2.67)	105 (2.55)	−5%
Gender			
Female	46 608 (97.33)	4 111 (99.69)	2%
Male	1 278 (2.66)	5 (0.30)	
Age bands			
< 20 years	68 (0.14)	9 (0.51)	72%
20–24 years	55 (0.11)	10 (0.51)	78%
25–29 years	221 (0.46)	56 (2.56)	82%
30–34 years	1 123 (2.34)	188 (6.14)	62%
35–39 years	2 036 (4.25)	445 (11.16)	62%
40–44 years	3 779 (7.89)	572 (14.74)	46%
45–49 years	4 360 (9.10)	1 138 (14.38)	37%
50–54 years	5 541 (11.57)	543 (12.23)	5%
55–59 years	6 271 (13.09)	355 (9.98)	−31%
6–64 years	6 108 (12.75)	279 (8.34)	−53%
65–69 years	5 973 (12.47)	205 (6.70)	−86%
70–74 years	5 576 (11.64)	146 (5.47)	−113%
75–79 years	3 831 (8.00)	96 (3.89)	−106%
8–84 years	1 960 (4.09)	46 (2.09)	−95%
85 years+	984 (2.054)	28 (1.22)	−67%
Province			
Eastern Cape (EC)	2 593 (5.41)	270 (8.96)	40%
Free State (FS)	1 677 (3.50)	152 (6.09)	43%
Gauteng (GP)	19 821 (41.39)	1 344 (32.46)	−28%
KwaZulu Natal (KZN)	5 838 (12.19)	702 (17.46)	30%
Limpopo (LP)	2 195 (4.58)	542 (4.30)	−7%
Mpumalanga (MP)	1 718 (3.58)	340 (6.70)	47%
Northern Cape (NC)	658 (1.37)	55 (2.66)	48%
North West (NW)	3 290 (6.87)	322 (5.73)	−20%
Not classified	205 (0.42)	12 (0.61)	30%
Outside South Africa	11 (0.02)	5 (0.25)	91%
Western Cape (WC)	9 880 (20.63)	372 (14.74)	−40%

	Cancer of the breast (N = 47,886) n (%)	Cancer of the cervix (N = 4,116) n (%)	% Difference
Hospital setting			
Out of Hospital (OOH)	32 891 (68.68)	2 109 (48.23)	−42%
In Hospital (IH)	14 995 (31.31)	2 007 (51.76)	40%

Table 4.
Demographic characteristics, number of beneficiaries (%).

8.1 Distribution of oncology specialists

Independent practice specialists' radio oncology services are available in all provinces. **Figures 5** and **6** show the distribution of oncology specialists by region. The results depict that many oncology specialists are concentrated in urban and more

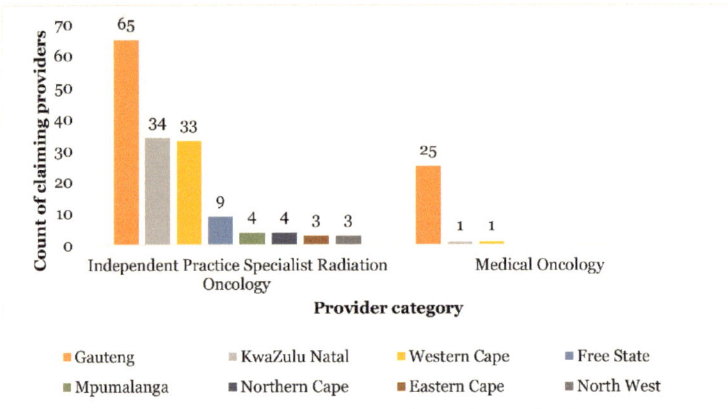

Figure 5.
Distribution of oncology specialists by province.

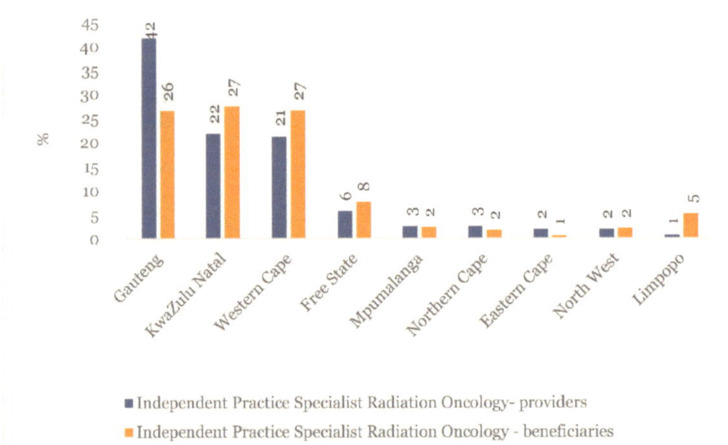

Figure 6.
Distribution of independent practice specialist radiation oncology providers by province- adjusted for utilising beneficiaries.

affluent areas such as Gauteng and KwaZulu Natal, as the proportion of providers was higher than that of beneficiaries within the province. Medical oncology services are based mainly in Gauteng province, which accounts for 92% of medical oncology services. At the same time, there are no medical oncology services in two regions, Western Cape and KwaZulu Natal, where each accounted for 4%. When adjusting for beneficiaries, there are significantly more independent practice specialists in radiation oncology than beneficiaries in Gauteng province. Slightly more beneficiaries than providers in KwaZulu Natal, Western Cape and the Free State province. There is a high scarcity of independent practice specialists in radiation oncology in Limpopo province, where the relative ratios were 1% vs 5%.

8.2 Benefits paid by setting

Table 5 shows benefits paid per beneficiary by setting. The average amount paid differed by setting. The average amount spent per beneficiary was nearly twice that in-hospital setting compared to the out-of-hospital setting, R53 680 vs R30 984 for breast cancer, respectively. Similarly, the average amount spent on cervical cancer was R54 760 vs R31 044 for in-hospital and out-of-hospital settings, respectively. On average, cervical cancer was more expensive (nearly R10 000 more) to treat than breast cancer, R46 905 vs R38 114. The maximum amount paid per beneficiary with cervical cancer was R523 695 and R962 103 out-of-hospital and in-hospital settings,

Setting	Cancer of breast	Cancer of cervix	Consolidated
Out of hospital	R30 985	R31 926	R31 044
In hospital	R53 680	R62 645	R54 760
	R38 114	R46 905	R38 827

Table 5.
Benefits paid per beneficiary by cancer type and setting.

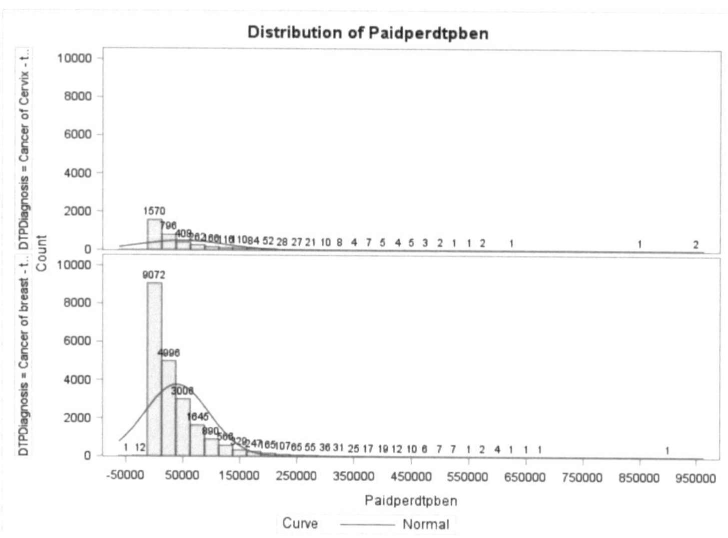

Figure 7.
Distribution of benefits paid per beneficiary (Cancer of the cervix and the breast).

respectively, as shown in **Figure** 7. The maximum amount paid per beneficiary for breast cancer was much higher for the in-hospital setting than for cancer of the cervix at R682 364. In contrast, the amount paid for breast cancer in the in-hospital setting was R 910 431.

8.3 Level of OOP by setting

Table 6 shows the levels of OOP by setting; the data indicate that the in hospital setting was twice that and out-of-hospital setting at 2 and 4% for breast cancer, respectively. The same phenomenon was notable in cervix cancer, where the OOP was 2% and 4% for out-of-hospital and in-hospital settings, respectively.

8.4 Benefits paid and OOP benefit design

The analysis of comprehensive and hospital plans attracted higher expenditure levels on cancer of the cervix at R57 205 and R53 037, respectively. However, for breast cancer, benefits paid per beneficiary were higher for EDOs and hospital plans at R42 740 and R41 797, respectively. Benefit design groupings further stratified the analysis. When adjusting for the funding of cancer of the breast, the data show higher levels of OOP in EDOs (5.3% OOP levels) and hospital plans (5.9% OOP levels) compared to comprehensive (3.3 % OOP levels) and partial cover type of plans (3.4% OOP level). A slightly different phenomenon emerges when adjusting for cancer of the cervix, where, hospital plans (4.9% of OOP levels), EDOs (3.8% of OOP levels) and partial cover plans (3.6% of OOP levels) accounted for higher levels of OOP compared to comprehensive plans (2.6% of OOP levels) (**Figure 8**).

Setting	Cancer of breast	Cancer of Cervix	Combined
Out of hospital	2%	2%	2%
In hospital	6%	4%	5%
	4%	3%	4%

Table 6.
Levels of OOP by setting.

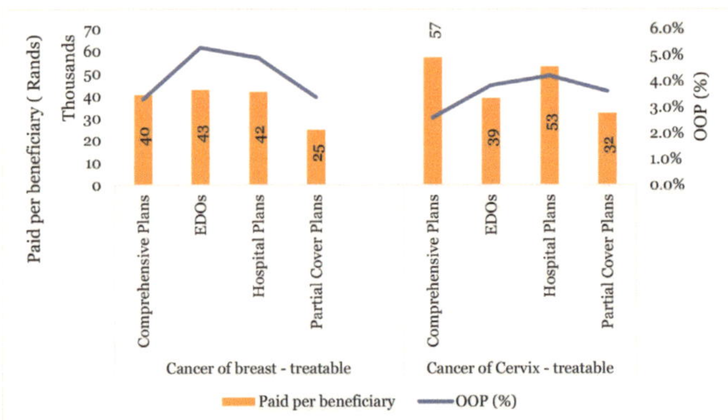

Figure 8.
Average amount paid per beneficiary and OOP levels by benefit design.

8.5 Scheme type: Sector

Table 7 shows that open scheme beneficiaries were exposed to slightly higher co-payment levels than those in restricted schemes. This was prevalent in both beneficiaries with cancer of the breast and those with cancer of the cervix. Similarly, with the average benefit paid on average, open schemes paid R41 797 for breast cancer compared to restricted schemes that paid R30 127. Again, open schemes paid even more for cervix cancer than restricted schemes, at R52 108 vs R43 160, respectively. Despite being less than 5%, OOP for open schemes was twice that of restricted schemes for cancer of the cervix beneficiaries, at 4% and 2%, respectively.

8.6 Scheme size

There were no significant differences in breast cancer funding by scheme size. The average expenditure per beneficiary for cervix cancer was higher for medium schemes at R57 911, followed by large schemes at R46 566 and small schemes at R42 176. However, large schemes paid slightly higher than medium and small schemes at R37 801, R35 713 and R30 733 per beneficiary for breast cancer, respectively (**Table 8**).

Scheme type	No of the DTP beneficiaries	Paid per DTP beneficiary	OOP (%)
Cancer of breast - treatable	47 886		
Open	30 111	R41 797	4%
Restricted	17 775	R30 127	3%
Cancer of Cervix - treatable	4 117		
Open	1 699	R52 108	4%
Restricted	2 418	R43 160	2%

Table 7.
Proportion of oncology benefits incurred by members by sector.

Scheme size	No of the DTP beneficiaries	Paid per DTP beneficiary	OOP (%)
Cancer of breast - treatable			
Large	44 912	R37 800,76	4%
Medium	1 978	R30 732,57	4%
Small	996	R35 713,29	3%
Cancer of Cervix-treatable			
Large	3 920	R46 565,81	3%
Medium	130	R57 911,83	4%
Small	67	R42 175,78	3%

Table 8.
Proportion of oncology benefits incurred by members by scheme size.

8.7 Multivariate regression analysis

Table 9 shows the results of the multivariate regression analysis; the results showed higher cervical cancer rates were significantly associated with the hospital setting, geographic distribution of beneficiaries, sector, and benefit design. At the same time, breast cancer was significantly associated with the geographical distribution of beneficiaries, sector, and scheme type. The odds ratio is 1.24, which indicates that the odds that the cervix's cancer rate was 1.24 times higher in an in hospital setting than in out-of-hospital. The odds ratio is 6.482, which suggests that the odds of higher rates of cancer of breast cancer are seven times higher in Gauteng than in Limpopo. The odd ratio of 8.521 indicated that the odds of higher rates were 9 times

Effect	Cancer of the cervix		Cancer of the breast	
	Odds ratio	95 % CI	Odds ratio	95 % CI
In Hospital 1 vs 0	1.24	(1.016, 1.514) *	1.038	(0.963, 1.118)
Province Code EC vs GP	2.508	(1.73, 3.636)	1.201	(1.041, 1.385)
Province Code FS vs GP	2.331	(1.513, 3.592)	1.19	(1.018, 1.391)
Province Code KZN vs GP	1.709	(1.283, 2.278)	1.06	(0.939, 1.195)
Province Code LP vs GP	6.482	(3.493, 12.026) **	1.077	(0.891, 1.301)
Province Code MP vs GP	2.097	(1.386, 3.171)	1.197	(1.017, 1.409)
Province Code NC vs GP	8.521	(3.83, 18.954) **	1.587	(1.286, 1.959) *
Province Code NW vs GP	3.415	(2.141, 5.446)	1.256	(1.064, 1.483)
Province Code OTH vs GP	0.577	(0.168, 1.982) *	1.191	(0.826, 1.718)
Province Code OUT vs GP	1.18	(0.17, 8.172)	0.548	(0.164, 1.825)
Province Code WC vs GP	2.313	(1.693, 3.161)	1.052	(0.943, 1.173)
Type Rest vs Open	1.494	(1.195, 1.868) **	1.165	(1.069, 1.269) *
Size Medium vs Large	0.01	(0.002, 0.042)	0.833	(0.737, 0.941)
Size Small vs Large	0.056	(0.026, 0.119)	0.89	(0.75, 1.057)
Benefit Design EDOs vs Comprehensive Plans	0.575	(0.408, 0.81)	0.98	(0.866, 1.109)
Benefit Design Hospital Plans vs Comprehensive Plans	1.594	(1.187, 2.141) **	0.99	(0.888, 1.104)
Benefit Design Partial Cover Plans vs Comprehensive Plans	0.769	(0.6, 0.985)	1.028	(0.933, 1.133)
Benefit Design Unknowns vs Comprehensive Plans	0.093	(0.043, 0.199) **	0.978	(0.812, 1.178)

*** $p < 0.001$; * $p < 0.05$; CI: Confidence Interval*

Table 9.
Multivariate logistic model assessing the association between demographic, scheme characteristics and setting variables as predictors of cancer proportion.

higher in Gauteng than in the Northern Cape. The cancer of the cervix was also significantly associated with scheme types. The odds ratio of 1.494 indicated that the odds of higher rates were nearly twice higher in open schemes than in restricted schemes. The results show the odds ratio of 1.165 for breast cancer, which indicated that the odds were nearly twice higher in open schemes than in restricted schemes. Similarly, North West, where the odds are 1.476, shows breast cancer rates are two times higher in Western Cape than in the Northern Cape province. Our study also found the effect of benefit design on the cervix's cancer rates, where the odds of 1.594 indicated that higher rates were in comprehensive plans than in hospital plans. The multivariate analysis results for breast cancer revealed that higher rates were significantly associated with the geographical distribution of beneficiaries in the Northern Cape and Gauteng provinces. The odds ratio of 1.587 indicated that Gauteng province had the odds of nearly twice higher rates than the Northern Cape province. The effect of the sector was also prevalent as this was statistically significant in both models. Benefit design and hospital setting did not affect the higher breast cancer rates.

9. Conclusion

This study finds a higher number of beneficiaries diagnosed with breast cancer, nearly ten times more than those diagnosed with cervix cancer. These findings are consistent with the literature, where breast cancer is the most common cancer in women [20–22, 27]. The study also found that 97% of breast cancer was diagnosed in females than in males, who accounted for 3 % of breast cancer, slightly higher than another study conducted in the public sector the study found the rate of 1.4% [33]. The findings, however, were still within range when compared to international norms ranging between 1–3% [29–31, 46]. The weighted average of women diagnosed with breast cancer was much older at 59 years; however, it was within the range of systematic review and meta-analysis, which showed the average age of female breast cancer in Africa ranged between 30.6 to 60.8 years [47]. There is evidence of a much younger mean age of beneficiaries diagnosed with cervical cancer. The findings of this study were consistent with a study conducted in the public sector in South Africa, which found a mean age of 56.2 years [33]. However, this study shows the early stage of diagnosis in medical schemes in the age band of 20–24 years, thus denoting risk exposure in much younger age profiles. The study found that cervix cancer was diagnosed ten years earlier than breast cancer, and the weighted average age of cervical cancer beneficiaries was 50 years. This is consistent with global trends reporting the average age range (50–53 years). Condition-specific findings show that the proportion of beneficiaries with breast and cervical cancer was higher in Gauteng (41% vs 33%). Though much lower, the Western Cape had a similar phenomenon where the proportion of breast cancer beneficiaries was more than twice that of cervical cancer beneficiaries (21% vs 9%). Other provinces showed a higher proportion of cervical cancer than breast cancer. The study discovered significant differences in the distribution of oncology specialists relative to covered lives in affluent urban provinces like Gauteng and Western Cape and rural provinces like the Eastern Cape and Limpopo. These disparities were more pronounced in KwaZulu Natal and Limpopo (17% vs 12% and 15% vs 5%), respectively. The Gauteng, Western Cape, and KwaZulu Natal provinces accounted for 85% of independent practice specialist oncologists, while the other provinces accounted for only 15%, with other provinces showing less than ten specialists. The distribution of oncologists was less represented in other provinces than Gauteng, which accounted for 93% of the claiming medical oncologists. The two other provinces (Western Cape and KwaZulu Natal) accounted for the balance, with only one medical oncology service provider each. In rural provinces, there was no claiming medical oncologist. These findings further describe higher inequalities geographically, which are also prevalent in the private sector. The study also found a higher proportion of covered lives relative to the balance of independent practice specialist radiation oncologists in Limpopo (Rural) at 1% vs 5%, depicting an urgent need to develop and attract specialists in the province. This finding conforms to previous studies (e.g., [7, 48]) in those urban residences increase the access and uptake of cancer screening. A study by van Eeden et al. [49] further confirmed challenges with oncology services for lung cancer, mainly radiotherapy units primarily located in larger cities, limiting access to rural-based areas. The implication of practical recommendations for medical schemes is a scarcity of medical service providers as they relate to designated service providers and specialist network contracting. The significant shortfall of oncology specialists in poorer provinces directly leads to long treatment delays. High patient volumes in this province affect optimal treatment care irrespective of the sector, as this study shows [50]. The findings revealed a relatively higher proportion of beneficiaries with breast cancer compared to cervical cancer beneficiaries in open schemes than in restricted schemes; in large schemes than in medium and small schemes; in comprehensive plans, EDOs, and hospital plans than in partial cover plans; and in age bands older than 55; in provinces such as the Gauteng, Limpopo, and North West and Western Cape provinces; and in out-of-hospital setting than in an in-hospital setting. The multivariate analysis further supported these findings, which found that higher cancer rates of cervical cancer were significantly associated with the hospital setting, geographic distribution of beneficiaries, sector, and benefit design. Furthermore, this study provides critical insights for the National Health Insurance as they address human resources and relative socio-economic challenges. The regression model's findings for breast cancer revealed that higher rates were significantly associated with the geographical distribution sector. The industry also affected the higher levels of cancer in the breast proportion. The odds ratio of 1.165 indicated that the odds were nearly twice as high in open schemes than in restricted schemes. Benefit design and hospital setting did not affect the higher breast cancer rates. The average expenditure for the two types of cancers differed by scheme type and was much higher in open schemes than in closed schemes, thus indicating the effect of setting. Cervical cancer was +/-R 10,000 more expensive than breast cancer per beneficiary. Partial cover plans paid around R25 000 for breast cancer compared to other benefit options, which paid around R40 000 per beneficiary region. EDOs and partial cover plans paid just under R40 000 for cervical cancer per beneficiary, while comprehensive and hospital plans paid just over R50 000. Finestone et al. [27] found that low-cost or less comprehensive benefit options paid much less for breast and cervical cancer treatments [27]. The authors found that the average cost for cervical cancer in the public sector ranged between R28 666 and R33 021 for stages 1–4.

The level of OOP for the two cancers was insignificant in the region of 2–4%; however, it still presents a financial burden to beneficiaries and could be detrimental for those rural-based provinces where the barrier to accessing specialist oncology services is even higher. The study recommends support programs (family support, government, medical service providers, private sector and government) for cancer patients and integrated into managed care services. Due to inequalities between and within the two-tiered health system in South Africa, the study proposes a multidisciplinary approach to address the scarcity of resources. Public-private partnerships on cancer treatment and support programs should be the critical feature to help move South Africa closer to Sustainable Development Goal (SDG) 3.4

To reduce, by one-third, premature mortality from NCDs+ through prevention and treatment and promote mental health and well-being by 2030 [51, 52].

10. Limitations

This study has the following methodological limitation:

- Expenditure per beneficiary did not distinguish between diagnosis and treatment (surgical and non-surgical), furthermore does not include additional and follow-up costs.
- Prevalence and incidence were not considered due to a lack of access to primary data
- The data do not consider the long-term treatment of the conditions analysed, including ongoing management of the diseases that could potentially have a cost implication.
- The study also did not adjust for the severity of the condition, nor did it consider demographic characteristics such as race which are potential risk factors.
- The study also did not consider co-morbidities which could exacerbate the conditions even further.

The analysis of the aggregated transaction data restricted the study because it did not consider patient or provider perspectives and experience; future studies should consider qualitative aspects such as patient experience. Future studies should include drivers of co-payment in PMB level of care conditions and an effort to develop approaches and interventions to minimise these.

Acknowledgements

The authors are grateful to Mr Phakamile Nkomo, Mr Martin Moabelo and Mr Sibusiso Ziqubu for their support in concluding this research work.

Conflict of interest

The authors declare that no financial or personal relationships may have influenced them inappropriately in writing this article.

Ethical considerations

The data were assessed and only reported at the consolidated level for privacy and confidentiality. No clinical or patient-specific information was accessed nor reported while conducting this research.

Author details

Michael Mncedisi Willie*, Thulisile Noutchang, Maninie Molatseli and Sipho Kabane
Council for Medical Schemes, Policy Research and Monitoring, Pretoria, South Africa

*Address all correspondence to: m.willie@medicalschemes.co.za

References

[1] Choi E, Lee YY, Suh M, Lee EY, Mai TTX, Ki M, et al. Socio-economic inequalities in cervical and breast cancer screening among women in Korea, 2005–2015. Yonsei Medical Journal. 2018;**9**:1026-1033

[2] Bruni L, Diaz M, Castellsagué X, Ferrer E, Bosch FX, de Sanjosé S. Cervical human papillomavirus prevalence in 5 continents: Meta-analysis of 1 million women with normal cytological findings. The Journal of Infectious Diseases. 2010;**202**:1789-1799

[3] Torre LA, Islami F, Siegel RL, Ward EM, Jemal A. Global cancer in women: Burden and trends. Cancer Epidemiology, Biomarkers & Prevention. 2017;**26**:444-457

[4] Ferlay J, Soerjomataram I, Dikshit R, Eser S, Mathers C, Rebelo M, et al. Cancer incidence and mortality worldwide: Sources, methods and major patterns in GLOBOCAN. 2012. International Journal of Cancer. 2015; **136**:E359-E386

[5] Swanson M, Ueda S, Chen LM, Huchko MJ, Nakisige C, Namugga J. Evidence-based improvisation: Facing the challenges of cervical cancer care in Uganda. Gynecologic Oncology Reports. 2018;**24**:30-35

[6] Hull R, Mbele M, Makhafola T, Hicks C, Wang SM, Reis RM, et al. Cervical cancer in low and middle-income countries. Oncololgy Letters. 2020;**20** (3):2058-2074

[7] Phaswana-Mafuya N, Peltzer K. Breast and cervical cancer screening prevalence and associated factors among women in the south african general population. Asian Pacific Journal of Cancer Prevention. 2018;**19**(6):1465-1470

[8] Moodley J, Constant D, Mwaka AD, Scott SE, Walter FM. Mapping awareness of breast and cervical cancer risk factors, symptoms and lay beliefs in Uganda and South Africa. PLoS ONE. 2020;**15**(10):e0240788

[9] Somdyala NIM, Bradshaw D, Dhansay MA, Stefan DC. Increasing cervical cancer incidence in rural eastern cape province of south africa from 1998 to 2012: A population-based cancer registry study. JCO Global Oncology. 2020;**6**:1-8

[10] Joffe M, Ayeni O, Norris SA, McCormack VA, Ruff P, Das I, et al. Barriers to early presentation of breast cancer among women in Soweto, South Africa. PLoS ONE. 2018;**13**(2):e0192071

[11] Goyal A, Gupta J, Choudhary A, Harit K, Ragesvari KS, Gupta I. Awareness about breast cancer in males in urban area of Delhi. Journal of Family Medicine and Primary Care. 2020;**9**(4): 1999-2001

[12] Isabirye A, Mbonye MK, Kwagala B. Predictors of cervical cancer screening uptake in two districts of Central Uganda. PLoS One. 2020;**15**(12): e0243281

[13] Torres KL, Rondon HHMF, Martins TR, Martins S, Ribeiro A, Raiol T, et al. Moving towards a strategy to accelerate cervical cancer elimination in a high-burden city-Lessons learned from the Amazon city of Manaus, Brazil. PLoS One. 2021;**16**(10):e0258539

[14] Kashyap N, Krishnan N, Kaur S, Ghai S. Risk factors of cervical cancer: A case-control study. Asia-Pacific Journal of Oncology Nursing. 2019;**6**(3): 308-314

[15] Shah SC, Kayamba V, Peek RM Jr, Heimburger D. Cancer control in low- and middle-income countries: Is it time to consider screening? Jornal of Global Oncololy. 2019;**5**:1-8

[16] World Health Orghanisation (WHO). Screening Programmes: A Short Guide Increase Effectiveness, Maximise Benefits and Minimise Harm. WHO. Screening Programmes: A Short Guide. Increase Effectiveness, Maximise Benefits And Minimise Harm. Copenhagen: WHO Regional Office for Europe; 2020

[17] Abratt, R. South African society of clinical and radiation oncology annual census Newsletter. 2020. [Internet]. Available from: http://sascro.org/wp-content/uploads/2015/12/sascro_newsletter24.pdf

[18] Ashmore J. 'Going private': A qualitative comparison of medical specialists' job satisfaction in the public and private sectors of South Africa. Human Resources of Health. 2013; **11**:1

[19] Icon. Icon Oncology drives sustainability of cancer care in South Africa. 2022. [Internet]. 2022. Available from: https://iconsa.co.za/2022/07/25/icon-oncology-drives-sustainability-of-cancer-care-in-south-africa/ [Accessed: August 22, 2022]

[20] Francies FZ, Hull R, Khanyile R, Dlamini Z. Breast cancer in low-middle income countries: Abnormality in splicing and lack of targeted treatment options. American Journal of Cancer Research. 2020;**10**(5):1568-1591

[21] Sung H, Ferlay J, Siegel RL, Laversanne M, Soerjomataram I, Jemal A, et al. Global cancer statistics 2020: GLOBOCAN estimates of incidence and mortality worldwide for 36 cancers in 185 countries. Cancer Journal for Clinicians. 2021 May;**71**(3):209-249

[22] Chitha W, Swartbooi B, Jafta Z, Funani I, Maake K, Hongoro D, et al. Model of delivery of cancer care in South Africa's Eastern Cape and Mpumalanga provinces: A situational analysis protocol. BMJ Open. 2022;**12**(2): e058377

[23] Ndlovu SR, Kuupiel D, Ginindza TG. Mapping evidence on the distribution of paediatric cancers in sub-Saharan Africa: A scoping review protocol. Systematic Reviews. 2019;**8**(1):262

[24] Lei S, Zheng R, Zhang S, Wang S, Chen R, Sun K, et al. Global patterns of breast cancer incidence and mortality: A population-based cancer registry data analysis from 2000 to 2020. Cancer Communication (Lond). 2021;**41**(11): 1183-1194

[25] Bahnassy AA, Abdellateif MS, Zekri AN. Cancer in Africa: Is It a Genetic or Environmental Health Problem? Frontiers in Oncology. 2020; **10**:604214

[26] Khalis M, Charbotel B, Chajès V, Rinaldi S, Moskal A, Biessy C, et al. Menstrual and reproductive factors and risk of breast cancer: A case-control study in the Fez region, Morocco. PLoS One. 2018;**13**(1):e0191333

[27] Finestone E, Wishnia J, Ranchod S. Estimating and projecting the burden of cancer in South Africa. Cancer Alliance. [Internet]. 2021. Available from: https://canceralliance.co.za/wp-content/uploads/2021/08/Percept-report-on-the-Cost-of-Cancer-in-South-Africa-v1.pdf

[28] Smolarz B, Nowak AZ, Romanowicz H. Breast cancer-epidemiology, classification, pathogenesis and

treatment (Review of Literature). Cancers (Basel). 2022;**14**(10):2569

[29] Madeira M, Mattar A, Passos RJ, Mora CD, Mamede LH, Kishino VH, et al. A case report of male breast cancer in a very young patient: What is changing? World Journal of Surgical Oncology. 2011;**9**:16

[30] Rayne S, Schnippel K, Thomson J, Reid J, Benn C. Male breast cancer has limited effect on survivor's perceptions of their own masculinity. American Journal of Men's Health. 2017;**11**(2): 246-252

[31] Khattab A, Kashyap S, Monga DK. Cancer, Male Breast Cancer. Treasure Island (FL): StatPearls Publishing; 2020

[32] Ndom P, Um G, Bell EM, Eloundou A, Hossain NM, Huo D. A meta-analysis of male breast cancer in Africa. Breast. 2012;**21**(3):237-241

[33] Kakudji BK et al. Epidemiological, clinical and diagnostic profile of breast cancer patients treated at Potchefstroom regional hospital, South Africa. 2012-2018: An open-cohort study. The Pan African Medical Journal. 2020;**36**:9

[34] Guzha NT et al. Development of a method to determine the cost of breast cancer treatment with chemotherapy at Groote Schuur Hospital, Cape Town. South Africa. South African Medical Journal. 2020;**110**(4):296-301

[35] Discovery Health Medical Scheme (DHMS). Top three cancers in South Africa, trends and costs according to Discovery Health Medical Scheme. 2020 [Internet]. 2020. Available from: https://www.fanews.co.za/article/company-news-results/1/discovery/1051/top-three-cancers-in-south-africa-trends-and-costs-according-to-discovery-health-medical-scheme/28240

[36] 1Life. How much does it cost to treat breast cancer? 2019 [Internet]. 2019. Available from: https://www.1life.co.za/blog/cost-treat-breast-cancer

[37] Akokuwebe ME, Idemudia ES, Lekulo AM, Motlogeloa OW. Determinants and levels of cervical Cancer screening uptake among women of reproductive age in South Africa: Evidence from South Africa Demographic and health survey data, 2016. BMC Public Health. 2021;**21**(1): 2013

[38] Arbyn M, Weiderpass E, Bruni L, de Sanjosé S, Saraiya M, Ferlay J, et al. Estimates of incidence and mortality of cervical cancer in 2018: A worldwide analysis. Lancet Global Health. 2022; **10**(1):e41

[39] Nyambe N, Hoover S, Pinder LF, Chibwesha CJ, Kapambwe S, Parham G, et al. Differences in cervical cancer screening knowledge and practices by HIV status and geographic location: Implication for program implementation in Zambia. African Journal of Reproductive Health. 2018; **22**(4):92-101

[40] Council for Medical Schemes (CMS). PMB Definition Guideline for Cervical Cancers. Council For Medical Schemes. Pretoria, South Africa: CMS

[41] Government Employees Medical Scheme (GEMS). Oncology management program. [Internet]. 2022. Available from: https://www.gems.gov.za/en/Healthcare-Programmes/Oncology-Management

[42] Platinum Health. Information guide. [Internet]. 2022. Available from: https://www.platinumhealth.co.za/wp-content/uploads/Platinum-Health-2021-Information-Guide-email-format.pdf

[43] Discovery Health Medical Scheme. Oncology program. [Internet]. 2022. Available from: https://www.discovery.co.za/wcm/discoverycoza/assets/medical-aid/benefit-information/2021/oncology-programme-2021.pdf

[44] Council for Medical Schemes Annual Report 2020/2021. Pretoria South Africa [Internet]. 2021. Available from: https://www.medicalschemes.co.za/annualreport2020/

[45] Nkomo PWF, Koch SF, Tshela EMM, Willie MM. Optimising beneficiary choices: Standardisation of medical scheme benefit options. South African Health Review. 2019;**2019**:90-104. Available from: https://www.hst.org.za/publications/Pages/SAHR2019.aspx. ISBN 978-1-928479-01-7

[46] Siegel RL, Miller KD, Jemal A. Cancer statistics, 2020. Cancer Journal for Clinicians. 2020;**70**(1): 7-30

[47] Adeloye D, Sowunmi OY, Jacobs W, et al. Estimating the incidence of breast cancer in Africa: A systematic review and meta-analysis. Journal of Global Health. 2018;**8**(1):010419

[48] Peltzer K, Phaswana-Mafuya N. Breast and cervical cancer screening and associated factors among older adult women in South Africa. Asian Pacific Journal of Cancer Prevention. 2014; **15**(6):2473-2476

[49] van Eeden R et al. Lung cancer in South Africa. Journal of Thoracic Oncology. 2020;**15**(1):22-28

[50] Sartorius K, Sartorius B, Govender PS, Sharma V, Sheriff A. The future cost of cancer in South Africa: An interdisciplinary cost management strategy. SAMJ: South African Medical Journal. 2016;**106**(10):949-950

[51] United Nations (UN). Transforming our world: The 2030 agenda for sustainable development. [Internet]. 2015. http://www.un.org/ga/search/view_doc.asp?symbol=A/RES/70/1&Lang=E [Accessed: July 16, 2022]

[52] Kroll C, Warchold A, Pradhan P. Sustainable Development Goals (SDGs): Are we successful in turning trade-offs into synergies? Palgrave Communications. 2019;**5**:140

Chapter 4

Healthcare Services for the Physically Challenged Persons in Africa: Challenges and Way Forward

Malik Olatunde Oduoye, Aymar Akilimali, Umulkhairah Arama, Mohammed Fathelrahman Adam, Uwezo Biamba Chrispin and Bonk Muhoza Gasambi

Abstract

This chapter is based on persons with physical disabilities in Africa, their challenges, and how it affects their health-seeking behaviors. We noticed that physical challenge has a substantial long-term adverse effect on one's ability to carry out normal day-to-day activities. Both the causes and the consequences of physical disability vary throughout the world, especially in Africa. Environmental, technical, and attitudinal barriers and consequent social exclusion reduce the opportunities for physically challenged persons to contribute productively to the household and the community and further increase the risk of falling into poverty and poor healthcare services. The inability of the physically challenged persons to perceive the lack of points of interest of government has intensified to make significant recommendations and possible solutions. This is appalling because the rate to which a community provides and funds restoration is a way of grading how much interest it has and the importance it connects to the quality of life of its citizens. We advocate and recommend swift actions and disability inclusiveness to accommodate persons with physical disabilities in Africa for them to have a good perception of life.

Keywords: physically challenged, persons, Africa, healthcare, services, way forward

1. Introduction

Disability is the interaction between the person with a medical condition (e.g., cerebral palsy, down syndrome, or depression) and personal and environmental factors (e.g., negative attitudes, inaccessible transportation and public buildings, and social support limit) [1]. Physical challenge has a substantial long-term adverse effect on one's ability to carry out normal day-to-day activities. Both the causes and the consequences of physical disability vary throughout the world, especially in Africa. Environmental, technical, and attitudinal barriers and consequent social exclusion

IntechOpen

reduce the opportunities for physically challenged persons to contribute productively to the household and the community and further increase the risk of falling into poverty and poor healthcare services.

The inability of the physically challenged persons to perceive the lack of points of interest of government has intensified to make significant recommendations and possible solutions. This is appalling because the rate to which a community provides and funds restoration is a way of grading how much interest it has and the importance it connects to the quality of life of its citizens. We also note that disability upsets the visions and habits of individuals because it is the pure manifestation of difference from a certain normality erected by social representations. We must allow those whom the chance of birth or life has placed in a situation of handicap, to be recognized as subjects and to fully play their role in society.

2. Concept of disability

2.1 Conceptual review

This concept is based on previous studies, articles, research, and paper reviews on persons with physical disabilities in Africa, their challenges, and how it affects their health-seeking behavior. We come to a realization that since the year 2001, the World Health Organization (WHO) has shown a wider, contemporary view of the concepts of "health" and "disability" through the recognition that every human being may encounter or have some degree of physical disability in their life span either through a change in health or environment. As you may know, physical disability is a global human experience, which is sometimes permanent and sometimes temporary. It is not something limited to a small part of the general population in the world [2]. Research shows that the number of people with disabilities has grown greatly over the last 2 decades. And it is estimated that there are over 1 billion disabled persons worldwide, with about 200 million of them experiencing very significant difficulties. This growth has been impacted both by the increasing life expectancy and by exposure to factors such as road traffic accidents, physical or mental stress, drug abuse, and infections. Thus, due to these factors mentioned, it is estimated that an individual born in a country where the mean life expectancy is 70 years of age is likely to spend, on average, 11 years of his/her life with some form of physical disability or challenge [1].

By definition, physical disability is a situation when there is a restriction in one's physiological functionality as well as anatomical activities, in other words, a person's day-to-day performances, movement, and flexibility (web.archive.org., 2003). This could be temporary, for a short period or long period, or may go into a lessening of the manifestations of the problems. Disability could be congenital or acquired. That is, a person could be born with physical disability from birth or after been born. The congenital disability could be due to some kind of genetic problems or chromosomal abnormalities. While the acquired form could be through external factors such as infections, harsh weather conditions, trauma, for example, road motor accidents. In a wide range, physical disability could exist. This could be from surgical removal of a limb (amputation), injury to the spinal cord, inflammation of the joints, progressive muscular weakness due to muscular dystrophy or from cerebral palsy, that is, a group of on-progressive, non-contagious conditions, caused by brain damage before birth or during infancy. Other conditions such as multiple sclerosis and Gullein–Barre syndrome have also been implicated.

Persons with physical disabilities are also human beings who form a proportionate size of population of the world in which they cannot be written off or neglected. According to research done by James et al., there are over 25 million individuals who have difficulty in moving around. This was made known by the National Coordinator of the Association of Indigenous People with Disabilities (AIPD), Dr. Josephy Ify Chikunie, a physically challenged lecturer at the University of Lagos (UNILAG), Akoka, Nigeria. Physically challenges have been seen to restrict the ability of an individual to perform excellently like other "abled" people as may be required. This is obvious to people through the ability to move or inability to move of the individual and thus can affect his or her ability to carry out habitual activities. In another way round, a physically challenged person is one who has a limitation with his body and, due to that, is unable to perform rudiment things that other people do easily. These rudiment things include but not limited to washing clothes, eating food, drinking water, sweeping, cycling, running, etc.

2.1.1 Prevalence of disability

We realized that the definition of disability, the quality and methods of data collection, rigor of sources, and varying disclosure rates are factors influencing the prevalence of disability. We also note that poor service provision and stigma may result in lower disclosure. On this note, we realized that national statistics can be misleading, incomparable, and inaccurate. And thus, these limitations may result in a higher prevalence of disability in developed countries being reported compared to developing countries. As a matter of fact, poor service provision, stigma, and predominantly collecting data through census result in lower-income countries recording lower disability prevalence rates compared to higher-income countries. Despite these potential influences, the data that do exist indicate that low- and middle-income countries in reality do have higher disability prevalence compared to high-income countries.

The prevalence of physical disability could also be enhanced by different factors many countries, most especially in sub-Saharan African countries. Certain features in health conditions, physical environmental factors, and other inconstant occurrences such as motor accidents, natural disasters, like earthquakes and volcanoes, a clash or disagreement, diet, and drug abuse, for example, cocaine, alcohol, has been identified. For example, an estimated 20 to 50 million people are injured by road motor accidents every year. And the number of people injured due to these accidents is not well documented, although road traffic injuries are estimated to account for about 1.7% of those living with physical disability. Also, individuals who have low source of livelihood, jobless, or have low educational background and stratification have been shown to have a higher risk of physical disability as compared with other children and those from poorer households, especially in the rural settlements, and have a significant higher burden of physical disability [3].

2.1.2 Global perspective

According to the WHO global disability action plan 2014–2021 [2]; globally, there is an estimate of over 1000 million people living with physical disability; this corresponds to 15% of the world's population or one in seven people. Among this population, between 110 million and 190 million adults experience significant difficulties in carrying out their normal physiological functions. A paper reviewed also showed an estimate of about 93 million children, and an equivalent of 1 in 20 of those below the age of 15 years, are living with a moderate or severe form of physical disability [4]. The number of people who experience physical challenges or disabilities will keep increasing as populations age, in a geometric form. Similarly, with the global increase in chronic health conditions, national patterns of disability are affected by certain trending features in health conditions and physical and social-environmental and other factors, such as road traffic injuries, falls, violence, emergencies including natural disasters, like earthquakes, volcanoes, and disagreements, unhealthy food and drinks and drug abuse [2].

2.1.3 Disability in Africa

According to the WHO, about 75% of people with disabilities are living in the developing countries. In Nigeria, for instance, WHO estimates put the number of people with disability at 19 million or approximately 20% of the country's population. Let us give a practical example. One of the authors of this chapter was discriminated by some of his lecturers in medical school in Nigeria, due to his impaired left arm. The author has untreated post-polio syndrome at the age 2 years, but was fortunate to study human medicine in the university. He was asked to change his medical course as a result of his impairment toward the end of his medical training. This made him frustrated and wanted to give up on his dream as a medical doctor.

Another scenario in the Eastern part of Nigeria, where a female medical doctor, named Dr. Judith Etim from the University of Nigeria, Nsukka (UNN), was discriminated due to her lower limb paralysis. Aside these sad stories and events, there are many untold stories of people in Africa with physical disabilities who have been discriminated and left to suffer. These people rather commit suicides if no one comes to their aid, or rather became beggar to sustain themselves. The question now is WHY? From the above stories, we realized that despite the expertise in therapeutic exercises and the available evidence of effectiveness, many people continue to live with physical disabilities across the globe, especially in Africa [5]. In Africa as in the world, people with physical disabilities face exclusion, discrimination, and difficulties in enjoying their rights, such as their rights to education, job, inheritance rights and property ownership, and social rights.

2.2 Information needs of the physically challenged persons in Africa

As we have highlighted earlier, persons with physical disabilities are also human beings like any other person; therefore, there are certain needs they long for. According to [6], these needs include the information for educational development and growth, the information needed for social and personal development, and the information needed for recreational or social purposes [3]. It must be emphasized that in trying to meet the above needs of persons living with physical challenges, in the library for instance, they are likely to need more assistance than the "abled" users.

We come to realize that it is also important that the information needs of the persons living with physical disabilities are quite numerous. Some of this information is available in the school libraries, music collections, spoken words collections, picture books, books in enlarged print, and high-interest/low-vocabulary materials. It is quite unfortunate that, in many countries in the world today, persons with physical disabilities still struggle to be educated/literate irrespective of their medical condition [3]. We realized that some of these people that are focused often perform better than their colleagues that are not suffering from any form of disabilities. For example, the case of one of the authors and Dr. Judith Etim. And after their education, the next thing they think of is how to get a befitting paid job [3].

3. Disability and accessing healthcare in Africa

According to the United Nations (UN) standard rules for equal opportunities (United Nations 1993), it is stated that having access to health and rehabilitation services is a vital condition to equal opportunities, and an important component of being a respected and productive member of the society [5]. Statically speaking, globally, about 15% of people with disabilities have difficulty accessing healthcare. These problems are particularly common among person with physically disability in Africa and most developing countries, and widen the access gap between them and their counterparts in the developed world. These challenges are compounded in low- and middle-income countries (LMICs) where factors such as poverty, poverty-related diseases, inefficient healthcare systems, training and equipment, inaccessible transportation systems, corruption, political instability, and negative attitudes toward disability occur. The combination of high needs and low capacity to pay for healthcare is a major policy concern and a serious global challenge for providing available, accessible, and affordable healthcare for person with physical disability. For each patient, access to care is a fundamental right. And for people with disabilities, the pathologies are more numerous.

People with a specific type of disability such as mental illness and intellectual or psychosocial disabilities often face high social exclusion. They consult later, present more frequent emergency situations and more complex problems, and are more difficult to reach by prevention campaigns. A study in Ghana reported that inaccessible healthcare facilities and equipment, specifically the absence of ramps and elevators, narrow corridors, the absence of toilets, and lack of sidewalks, were among the biggest barriers to access healthcare services. Each individual with disability should obtain appropriate healthcare services in situations of perceived need for care.

A study conducted among South Africans with disabilities shows that these healthcare challenges aggravate the existing health conditions in them. There exist many layers of injustice, unfairness, and bias, as a result of the era of policy of racial separation/segregation and discrimination, which further worsens the challenges of the persons with disabilities face every day. This study further revealed that despite the adoption of democracy in 1994, many African people with physical disabilities remain less privileged in many ways, with African physically challenged females facing more discrimination based on their ethnicity, tribe, gender, and physical disability. Also, this study made it clear that the challenges facing persons with disabilities living in rural communities are even worse due to the lack of healthcare services, medical experts, long distant travels, poor motorable roads, as well as high rate of stigmatization related to physical disability.

Furthermore, we realized that during times of hardship like times of disaster, and other unforeseen occurrences, many individuals with physical disabilities are further alienated and opted out. These individuals witness an inability to access basic healthcare services especially from the primary healthcare centers and secondary health facilities. They are faced with difficulties to obtain information in an accessible way and receive good medical evaluations and interventions. Also, with regard to the era of COVID-19 pandemic, more factors such as preexisting comorbidities, as well as public living spaces like the home or educational facilities, further make the individuals with physical challenge vulnerable to contract the COVID-19 virus [3]. Many have also experienced struggle and direct discrimination in accessing life-saving treatment such as critical care admission, ICU, and oxygen support. We believed that some of these issues have made persons with physical challenges more susceptible to a higher risk of contracting the COVID-19 virus during the present pandemic era.

Overall, persons with physical challenges have problems to have the possibility to identify healthcare needs, to seek healthcare services, to reach the healthcare resources, to obtain or use healthcare services, and to actually be offered services appropriate to the needs for care. They could not conceptualize five dimensions of accessibility of service, such as approachability, acceptability, availability and accommodation, affordability, and appropriateness.

3.1 Problems to means of transportation for healthcare services

Generally speaking, Africans have problems in accessing good transportation. These problems are compounded with people living with disabilities, most especially in seeking for healthcare. In Nigeria, for example, most of the roads are dilapidated. Most "abled" individuals are even finding it difficult to drive on these bad roads not to talk of the physically challenged people. As a result of this, most people living with disabilities in Africa and other developing countries find it difficult to go to the nearest hospitals for help. Thus, imposing their problems simultaneously and consequently, they develop more complications either from road accident or the disease itself. Similarly, most railway networks in many African countries are not accessible to wheelchair users. Unfortunately, there are limited or no assistance or support given to assist passengers with physical challenge in accessing and using trains. This makes these passengers more vulnerable because of safety concerns and measures.

In addition, several studies have shown that many African countries do not have telecoil (TTY) facilities available for passengers using hearing aids, and many airport stations have bad signage and faulty audio speaker devices. Persons with physical disabilities in many African countries experience many challenges, including lack of assistance getting into and out of a taxi. Most of these people are required to lift and carry their own wheelchairs on board, being charged an extra fare for their wheelchairs and concerns surrounding safety. In South Africa, for example, during national COVID-19 pandemic lockdown Level 1 and Level 2, public transport was significantly reduced in order to assist in containing the spread of the COVID-19 virus. Public train transportation was suspended, a limited number of busses were permitted, and small bus taxis were allowed to operate at limited capacity for limited hours. Transport was allowed for health professionals and other workers employed in essential work space and services, and individuals that require basic life amenities such as food, clothing, and shelter.

In recent times, it is quite unfortunate and sad in many African countries that travel time limits were too confined for many persons with physical challenges as a result of their disabilities and dependence on assistance and or support from others, requiring a longer time to finish up their morning hygiene routine, travel to buy food and medical provisions, and return home. It is of this note that the limited public transportation intensely affected the ability of caregivers to travel to assist the persons living with physical disabilities [7].

3.2 Problem for means of personal assistance and caregivers

It has been shown that persons with physical disabilities as well as their relatives carried an inner and incessant fear that their caregivers may be susceptible to sickness and/or need to be isolated [4]. Unlike high-income African countries such as Rwanda, Ghana, Nigeria, and South Africa where caregivers are paid for or procured *via* government structures and agencies [2], South Africans with disabilities are obligated to pay for caregivers in reserved way or use their R1890 state disability grant for this means. Also, we realized that in most cases, caregivers travel on public transport and interact with others at home, socially and while shopping when not on duty. Loneliness and social isolation from caregivers have also been shown to affect some persons with physical challenges and could have a long-term detrimental impact on their psychomotive well-being. It has been reported that isolation from caregivers who assist with drugs, together with reduced accessibility to mental health services, could lead to relapse of the disease [4, 7].

3.3 Problems with communication systems

Many African countries have poor communication systems. These are worse with persons with physical disabilities. The people living with hearing difficulties have limited accessible to hearing aids and interpretations. Studies show that African healthcare policy dictates that patients living with disabilities may not be followed by their friends or family when accessing healthcare, as these could impose more communication barriers and challenges to these people [7]. It is obvious that many deaf persons use sign language as their primary methods of communication and are unable to communicate with healthcare workers without interpretation. Also, for individuals who rely on lip reading, understanding healthcare workers wearing medical masks is not possible. Furthermore, we realized that the provision of a patient with disability history or having to sign consent may pose an obstacle, at times not possible for an individual with severe mental or psychosocial disabilities, or on the autistic symptoms [8].

3.4 Problems for means of curative management, restoration, and medications

Generally speaking, many countries face restorative solutions to disability problems especially chronic forms of disabilities and those that are related to nervous system. These problems are more rampant in most African tertiary healthcare facilities. Most of these facilities do not have a sophisticated physical therapy facilities to restore physical disabilities as well as well-trained experts in that aspect of medicine. Thus, many people with physical disabilities in Africa would rather have a sequela of their disabilities or die like that in their disabled form. Although African countries such as Nigeria, Ghana, South Africa, Rwanda, and Egypt have tried to establish neurophysiotherapy and functional recovery centers to correct some physical disabilities due to stroke, cerebral palsy, poliomyelitis, etc., only a few successes have been recorded. We realized that most of these centers end up referring their patients with such debilitating and physical impairment to the Western countries for possible curative and restoration, such as limb lengthening, nerve grafting, tendon transfer surgeries, and prosthetic insertions.

3.5 Problems in accessing intensive care and emergency management and triage

Several studies on emergencies and disasters show that when availability of resources is restricted, healthcare workers may be forced to make decisions as to who qualifies to receive life-saving healthcare. In emergency situations, such as the World

Trade Centre attack (2001), and natural disasters such as earthquakes and hurricanes, the significance of having triage policies in place and what challenges that can occur if they are not established in emergency situations arises. For example, most hospitals, nowadays, adopt the Advanced Trauma Life Support (ATLS) system in managing multiple injured patients as well as mass casualties [9].

Triage policies are important in normalizing the allocation of resources and care, as well as guiding healthcare workers in emergency practice. There are different methods of triage systems utilized across the globe and are different within countries that have dual healthcare systems; for example, the scoop and run system is mostly practiced in many African healthcare systems, for example, in Ahmadu Bello University Teaching Hospital (ABUTH), Shika, Kaduna state, Nigeria, the University of Ilorin Teaching Hospital (UITH), Ilorin, Kwara state, Nigeria, and the University College Hospital (UCH), Ibadan, Oyo state, Nigeria. Unfortunately, even though this is been practiced, there are no special arrangements and inclusiveness to accommodate persons living with disabilities.

While triage policies are fundamental to effective emergency healthcare services, it is important to ensure that they do not discriminate against any specific population group especially with persons living with physical disabilities. We realized that such discrimination is currently in practiced in London, UK (United Kingdom), where, during the COVID-19 pandemic, persons with physical disabilities and the less privileged persons have reportedly been denied the rights to be admitted into health centers or receive life-saving emergency treatment if they become sick [7].

4. Challenges of physically challenged persons in Africa

We realized that disability affects virtually everybody but more rampant among the women, children, older people, and poor people in different proportions. African children from poorer homes, indigenous populations, and those in ethnic minority groups are significantly higher risk of experiencing disability. Women and girls with disability are likely to experience what is called double discrimination. Double discrimination as a concept includes gender-based violence, abuse, marginalization, and stereotyping. As a result, women with disabilities are likely to face more disadvantages when compared to men with physical challenges and women without physical challenges. A country man, internally displaced, or stateless persons, refugees, migrants, and prisoners with physical challenge also face peculiar problems [10].

4.1 Challenges in the health sector

The relationship between poor health and disability is not fully understood. However, persons with disabilities are commonly poorer, and suffer from stigmatization and discrimination in education, employment and access to different services [1]. We noticed that the challenges faced by disabled persons in accessing healthcare are not new and are numerous. Physically disabled persons have always been faced with challenges in healthcare services, political or leadership positions, and education. According to MacLachlan and Mannan [1], access to healthcare, even in wealthy countries, is often difficult for persons with disabilities, but in poorer countries the challenges are exacerbated, combining physical, financial, and attitudinal components. Many policies have been put in place to improve these people's access to healthcare, but until now, physically disabled people show worse health outcomes than others. In addition to poor health system infrastructure and poor healthcare services in African countries, the access to healthcare services by persons with disabilities remain an unsolved challenge [2]; for example, in South Africa, persons with disabilities were found to have a higher un approached health needs compared to persons without disabilities [5].

There are many factors that serve as barriers to access healthcare services for persons with disabilities in Africa which include (1) stigmatization, (2) negative attitudes toward physically disabled persons, (3) cost of access to healthcare services and insufficient resources as a result of unemployment and poverty, (4) inadequate policy implementations by health and political authority, (5) physical inaccessibility to healthcare services, (6) long distance of health facilities and lack of transportation, (7) insecurity, (8) hilly terrains and flooding of rivers during the rainy season, (9) challenges as a result of inadequately trained healthcare providers to deal with disabled persons including poor communication and poor attitude, and (10) gender-based challenges in which women were the most affected group [3, 5, 7].

Those challenges commonly increased along with disability severity, being female in gender and declined with increasing education level, type of household, and age [2, 5]. Furthermore, in Africa, many physically challenged people are neglected because many of them are in the lower class in society, and many are left with no one to cater to them. They are often only catered to by their family members and sometimes neglected by the government. It is no doubt that many African countries are low-income countries, and healthcare systems are less developed compared with other countries in the world. A study conducted by Vergunst et al. [2] in rural Madwaleni, South Africa, showed that physically disabled persons faced barriers in accessing healthcare services, and the widely faced barrier was transportation; meanwhile, a higher level of education and socioeconomic status often reduced those barriers [11]. Another challenge is the sentiments and stereotypes toward people with disabilities. Some people view disabilities as punishments and abnormalities. A study conducted by Haruna [5] in Tamale Metropolis, Ghana, showed that some of the barriers faced by physically disabled people include the following: (1) sociocultural factors that consist of variables such as education, ignorance, stigmatization, and belief systems that exist within households and the communities, (2) service factors that relate to conditions prevailing at the health facility are the attitude of providers, service cost, waiting times, insurance, and distance, and (3) economic factors relating to income, occupation, and transport cost determine the physically disabled person's ability to access health services. Consequently, the falling standard of healthcare systems and migration of healthcare workers from African countries have worsened access to healthcare for physically disabled people. The lack of infrastructures like roads and standard hospitals, and lack of adequate policies that improve the welfare and inclusion of physically disabled people have increased the inaccessibility of physically disabled people to healthcare [10].

5. Recommendations and way forward

To address this issue, in which we believe stigma and the autonomy of people with disabilities are heavily implicated, we recommend to the African and international communities to think carefully about the psychological and social repercussions suffered by disabled people who have difficulty accessing care, and to integrate into humanitarian aid programs a space reserved for supporting both financially and in terms of education for the independence of people with disabilities. This includes: (1)—To encourage initiatives, among others: investments, candidacies,... by people with disabilities in all sectors of activity. (2)—The establishment of specific organizations to support people with disabilities in terms of health and easy access to care [2]. To African governments to subsidize health insurance for all persons physically unable to work, (3)—to set up specialized structures at each medical training course for easy and unlimited access to care for any disabled person [2]. To sensitize the African population in the fight against discrimination or all other forms of stigmatization and to call on them to work together in perfect cohabitation... [5]. To nursing staff—to administer equal and satisfactory treatment to everyone. Taking for instance, the case of South-African government policy [5].

In a nutshell, we are recommending disability inclusiveness for persons with disabilities and anti-discrimination policies from the all-African government. We believed that this policy would provide an important backdrop to the development of more inclusive health services for persons with disabilities in Africa. As this would also reflect a greater understanding and awareness of the experience of individuals with disabilities in their health-seeking behaviors and of the impact of disabling barriers on their independence, and strengthening their autonomy, health and well-being, as a result, health service providers in African countries would be able to address the issues of medical consultation with and participation of persons with disability in planning and quality healthcare service delivery [12].

6. Conclusion

Persons with physical challenges in African countries experience significant challenges especially in having quality healthcare services and support. Most of these people are denied their rights to seek good and affordable healthcare and restorative services. They are often left to suffer in pain, frustrations, and regrets. Injustice, marginalization, and inequality have made them to have bad perceptions about a good quality of life. Thus, we are advocating for full inclusion of persons with disabilities. Anti-discrimination has provided an important backdrop to the development of more inclusive health services for persons with disabilities.

Acknowledgements

We give thanks to the Almighty God for giving us the abilities to put this piece of writing together. Special thanks to the main author of this book, Mr. Malik Olatunde Oduoye, who corroborated with us from different parts of Africa. We are indeed grateful. We also acknowledged our parents, siblings, teachers, friends, and colleagues for their support in helping us with ideas, and moral and financial supports. We say a big thank you to all of you.

Funding is by all authors that contributed to this book.

Conflict of interest

The authors declare no conflict of interest.

Dedications

We dedicate this chapter to all persons living with physical challenges and disabilities in Africa.

Notes/thanks/other declarations

We declare that this chapter is for people who have interest in disabilities and willing to help and support people living with disabilities in the world, especially in Africa. Thank you all and God bless you! Amen!

Acronyms and abbreviations

WHO	World Health Organization
QoL	Quality of Life
ICU	Intensive Care Unit
UK	United Kingdom
USA	United States of America
UNESCO	United Nations Educational, Scientific and Cultural Organization
ILO	International Labour Organization
YLD	Years lived with Disability
DALYs	Disability-adjusted life Years

Author details

Malik Olatunde Oduoye[1*], Aymar Akilimali[2], Umulkhairah Arama[1], Mohammed Fathelrahman Adam[3], Uwezo Biamba Chrispin[4] and Bonk Muhoza Gasambi[2]

1 Ahmadu Bello University, Zaria, Kaduna State, Nigeria

2 Faculty of Medicine, Official University of Bukavu, Bukavu, Democratic Republic of Congo

3 University of Science and Technology, Omdurman, Sudan

4 Universite de Goma, Goma, Democratic Republic of Congo

*Address all correspondence to: malikolatunde36@gmail.com

References

[1] OMS. Handicap et santé. World Health Organization (WHO). 2021. pp. 1-1. Available from: https://www.who.int/news-room/fact-sheets/detail/disability-and-health

[2] World Health Organization (WHO). WHO Global Disability Action Plan 2014-2021. Better Health for all People with Disability. Switzerland: World Health Organization (WHO); 2015. pp. 1-32

[3] Idhalama OU. Provision of reference and information services to the physically challenged persons In Nigeria: Challenges and prospects. 2018. pp. 1-20. Available from: https://www.researchgate.net/publication/332495531

[4] United Nations - Division for Social Policy Development (DSPD D of E and SA (DESA). Toolkit on Disability for Africa - Disability-Inclusive Development. 2012. pp. 1-36. Available from: https://www.un.org/development/desa/dspd/2016/11/toolkit-on-disability-for-africa-2/

[5] Program GE, Hills T, Centre H, Hills T. Disability Care in Nigeria : The need for professional advocacy. 2009;30-36

[6] Egunjobi RA. Towards Meeting the Library and Information Needs of the Handicapped in Nigeria. In: Adedoja TA, Ajobiewe T, editors. Issues in Coping with Disability. 2003. p. 205

[7] McKinney EL, McKinney V, Swartz L. Access to healthcare for people with disabilities in South Africa: Bad at any time, worse during COVID-19? South African Family Practice. 2021;**63**(1):a5226. DOI: 10.4102/safp.v63i1.5226

[8] Vankova D, Mancheva P. Quality of life of individuals with disabilities. Scripta Scientifica Salutis Publicae 2015;**1**(1):21-28

[9] Love B A Short Practice Textbook of Surgery. 26th ed. 2015:1-1000

[10] Bright TKHA. Systematic review of access to general healthcare services for people with disabilities in low- and middle-income countries. International Journal of Environmental Research and Public Health. 2018. pp. 1-15

[11] Vergunst R, Swartz L, Hem KG, Eide AH, Mannan H, MacLachlan M, et al. Access to health care for persons with disabilities in rural South Africa. BMC Health Services Research. 2017;**17**:1-8

[12] United Nations-Division for social Policy Development (DSPD D of E and SA (DESA). Inclusive Health Services for Persons with Disabilities. Washington DC: United States of America (USA); 2012. pp. 1-37

Chapter 5

The Urgency of Access to Men-Centered Mental Healthcare Services to Address Men's Sensitive Issues in the Communities of South Africa

Mxolisi Welcome Ngwenya and Gsakani Olivia Sumbane

Abstract

South Africa yet again faces an upsurge of a national crisis. Approximately 13,774 deaths were reported in 2019 as a result of suicide. In total, 10,861 of the deaths were men. It has been said men usually take time to seek healthcare services. Most regard their problems to be solved over a few bottles of alcohol. Most of the suicides are linked to mental health issues. This poses an inquiry on the current services offered to address men's mental health issues. Therefore, this shows the significant urgency to access modified men-centered mental health services to address men's sensitive issues in the communities of South Africa (SA). However, this chapter seeks to review the prevalence of suicides, health-seeking behavior among men, and factors to poor utilization of mental health services in men. In addition, it discusses the proposed strategies to improve access to men-centered mental healthcare services.

Keywords: access, men-centered, mental healthcare, suicide, coping mechanisms

1. Introduction

Mental health is the state of which one is aware of self, able cope with normal stress situations, and work productively. However, some studies define mental health as a state of which there is absence of mental illness [1, 2]. South Africa yet faces an upsurge of national crisis of men's death in relation to mental health problems. Approximately 13,774 deaths were reported in 2019 because of mental-health-related problems. In total, 10,861 of the deaths were men. It has been said men usually take time to seek mental healthcare services. Most men regard problems to be solved over few bottles of alcohol. Studies showed that men have been found to seek psychological help at a lower rate compared to women [3, 4].

Men are more at risk of dying of suicide than women in South Africa. When compared with 10 years ago, more men are found to be depressed and are being admitted to psychiatric hospitals due to burnout and depression [5]. The Depression and Anxiety Group affirmed that men do not seek help until later when it is more serious, and although depression is ranked high on the list of chronic diseases, most men are not on treatment. The risk factors for mental health illness in men in South Africa are alcohol, substance use, unsafe sexual practice, diet, lack of physical exercises, violence, and other stressful life events [5].

Based on the recent statistics on suicide rates, it seems as if men's mental health is being neglected. It is against this background for the urgency of access of men-centered mental healthcare services to address men's sensitive issues in the communities of South Africa. Therefore, it requires redirection of resources to achieve a 100% sustainable mental health for all through access to men-oriented mental healthcare services to address sensitive issues among men.

2. Prevalence of suicides associated with mental health issues among men

Mental health is of significance to the well-being of individuals. However, individuals go through events in life that cause stress altering the mental health, consequently, resulting into suicides. Suicide is a major health problem worldwide contributing to 1.4% of the mortalities. The majority of the suicides are associated with mental health problems [6]. Over the years, gradual increase in acknowledgement of the role mental health in individual lives has been noted. Despite this progress and the transformed health system, men die every day as a result of mental health issues. Suicide is one of the leading causes. Furthermore, nearly 40% of countries have greater than 15 suicide deaths per 100,000 men [3, 7], with Lesotho, Guyana, Eswatini, South Korea, and Russia being the highest. Over 3000 Australians died of suicide every year. Some studies affirmed that majority of the suicides are linked mental illness such as depression, psychosis, and substance use [3].

Suicide is the twelfth leading cause of death in the United States, approximately 45,979 Americans died in 2020 as a result of suicide, and 1.2 million suicide attempts were reported. Correspondingly majority of the suicides were men accounting for 69.68%. Furthermore, in 2020, mortalities of men who died of suicide were 3.88 times than women [8]. The suicide rates have been gradually increasing over the years [9]. Similarly, in Shanghai, China, a rise in deaths due to suicide was noted, and most of the deaths were men with a rate of 6.38 per 100,000. Moreover, 22.54% of the suicide deaths were due to depression [10]. However, there are other factors associated with suicides; this includes sociodemographic, physical, lifestyle, stressful life events, and mental health factors (**Figure 1**) [11].

South Korea is the fourth highest country with higher suicides at a suicide rate of 28.6 per 100,000 [3]. Majority of the suicides were men with a suicide rate of 35.5

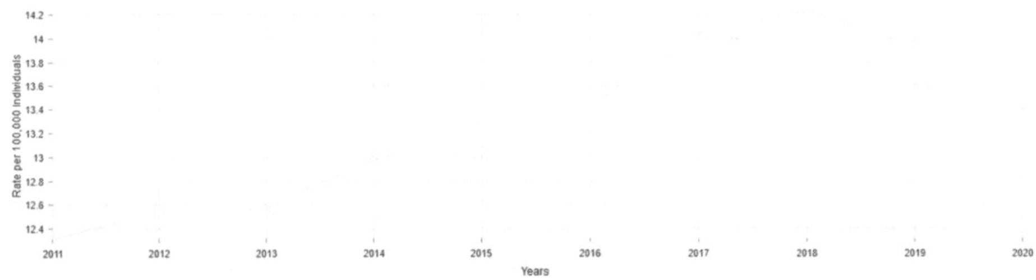

Figure 1.
Shows the rates of suicide in the United States over the years [9].

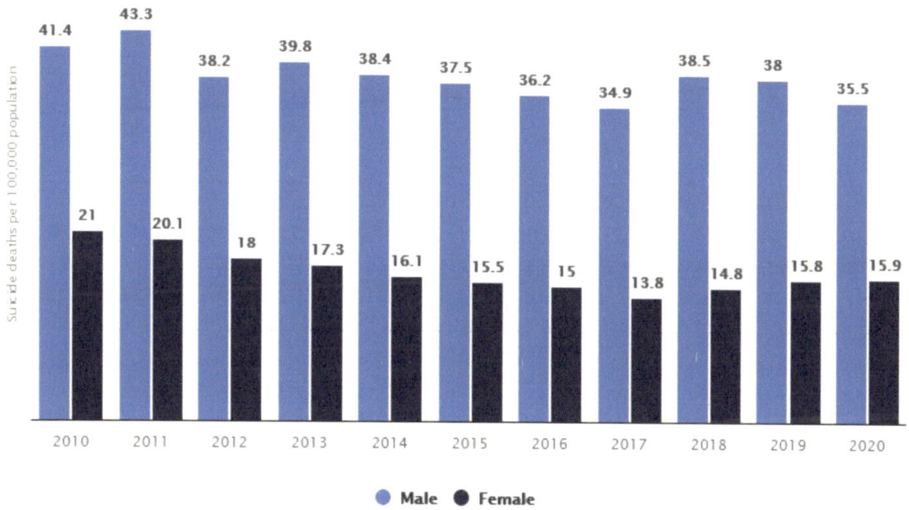

Figure 2.
Shows number of suicide deaths in South Korea by gender per 100,000 [14].

per 100,000 deaths being the third highest suicide rate globally. It was revealed that some of the suicides were due to social factors, religious activities, and higher social isolation [3, 12]. However, the state of health reported that the reasons for committing suicides among Koreans were mental illness, which accounted for the 28% of the men, and financial problems as well as physical illness [13]. Therefore, this shows the significant urgent need of mental health services for men (**Figure 2**).

Suicidal behavior is a major public health concern global and in Africa. Studies in Africa revealed that suicide rates in Africa are three times higher in men than women [15, 16]. In South Africa, the suicide rates are approximately five times in men than women. As of 2012, suicides rates ranged from 11.5 per 100,000 to as high as 23.5 per 100,000 in 2019, rendering South Africa being number tenth of the countries with highest suicide rates [3, 17]. An exploratory study on how group of young South African men think and talk about suicide revealed that they perceived suicide as goal-directed behavior that provides a means of recuperating control, asserting power, communicating and rendering oneself being noticeable [18].

3. Major mental health conditions associated with suicide in men

A number of studies have specified that there is silent crisis in men's health, which is mental health. Over the years, the number of suicides linked to mental health conditions has been gradually increasing. Most studies affirmed that the most common mental health conditions among men subsequently resulting in suicide were depression, anxiety disorders, and substance abuse [6, 19]. Here below only depression is discussed as it is the major ignored one among men.

3.1 Depression

Over the years, depression has been positioned as a mental health disorder dominant in women. However, changes have been observed over the years where more males are affected by depression; it been said some of the causes include financial problems, family problems, and overwhelming family responsibilities [20, 21]. Depression is regarded as an illness in which it affects the cognitive behavior of individuals. It affects how one thinks, feels, and acts [21]. Approximately 6 million men are affected by depression in the United States. Most of the men suffering from depression often remain undiagnosed or untreated, consequently resulting into suicide. Men's mental health has persisted undertheorized. One of the reasons includes social norms and masculinity such as statements like "Boys don't cry and men don't shed a tear." [22–24]. Furthermore, various masculinities identities and roles are implicated by men's depression; for instance, men's depression can be of result of divorce whereby the men are disrupted of from provider and protector roles. Moreover, also unemployment can exacerbate or trigger depression [25]. However, signs and symptoms of depression do not differ between males and females. Most depressed individuals exhibit different signs and symptoms, this includes [26]:

- Depressed mood all day, sometimes every day, i.e., feeling of sadness, empty, or hopelessness.
- Diminished interest or pleasure to all activities.
- Weight loss not related to diet
- Insomnia or hypersomnia almost everyday
- Fatigue or loss of energy nearly everyday
- Feelings of worthlessness nearly everyday
- Diminished ability to think, concentrate, or indecisiveness
- Recurrent thoughts of death

4. Factors contributing to poor access to mental healthcare in men

4.1 Role of culture

The role of culture in mental health is not well understood in spite of the fact that the cultural conception of the self has a powerful influence on the manner in which the disorder is expressed and understood. The majority of men's understanding of mental disorder is informed by an indigenous cultural perspective. Men make sense of their illness from both cultural perspective and social context in which they found themselves. Some men's understanding of mental disorder is in terms of issues such as witchcraft [27].

4.2 Socialization into traditional masculine gender roles

Men are thought to be deterred from engaging in mental health services due to socialization into traditional masculine gender roles. The social and cultural expectations make men think of themselves as risk-takers, thus leading to the probability of engaging more in risky behaviors that could lead to injury and death. Environmental pressures have been proposed to be one of the major causes of men's premature death and have predisposed them to engage in unhealthy behaviors (e.g., risky sexual behavior, alcohol use and abuse, high-risk sports, reckless driving) detrimental to their mental health. The chances that men will seek mental health when they feel discomfort are reduced because of their socialization experiences.

Men are often socialized through role-playing in such a way that they undermine help-seeking behavior, and if at all they intend to seek help, the individual is faced with cognitive dissonance, which is a consequence of contradictory beliefs of what they believe they are and what action they intend to take. Traits associated with traditional masculinity include stereotypes of stoicism, invulnerability, and self-reliance, which are frequently discussed as they do not fit comfortably with psychological help-seeking. For instance, negative emotions are perceived as a sign of weakness, discouraging men from reaching out to friends. This negatively impacts men's overall help-seeking behaviors and their choice of treatment type. Failure to adhere to these masculine stereotypes can result in the internalization of discriminative views held by the wider public. These self-stigmatizing beliefs further discourage men from seeking help [28, 29].

4.3 The problem of stigma – Social rejection and labelling

Stigma is described as a painful and distressing experience and a significant barrier to the inclusion of persons living with mental disorders in community activities, healthcare service, workplaces, and accessing education [27].

4.4 Differences in coping strategies

Men cope with mental health difficulties differently compared to women, demonstrating an increased tendency to self-medicate with alcohol and drugs to alleviate emotional distress.

4.5 Poor mental health

Literacy is reported to be associated with lower use of mental health services. Men are regarded as having poorer mental health literacy compared to women as they are worse at identifying mental health disorders [27].

4.6 Lack of appropriate diagnostic instruments and clinician biases

Men express symptoms of depression that do not always conform to the Diagnostic and Statistical Manual of Mental Disorders [30]. For example, they may express more externalizing behaviors such as alcohol consumption, irritability, and aggressive behaviors while underreporting other symptoms. These factors may mask men's difficulties, leading to inaccurate diagnoses and inappropriate treatment.

4.7 Clinicians may suffer from their own biases with the expectation that men should fulfill particular masculine stereotypes

For example, when men do not conform to these traditional masculine stereotypes by expressing themselves emotionally or by taking responsibility for their health, they may be regarded as deviant and/or feminine. These biases influence the quality and type of care provided and leave men less likely to receive a diagnosis despite presenting with similar or identical symptoms to women [29].

5. Adverse coping strategies used by men to deal with mental health-sensitive issues

5.1 Substance abuse

Substance use and mental health issues have substantial impact on individuals, families, communities, and societies [31]. Substance abuse is often linked to a number of triggering factors and to deal with such factors, men often resort to substance use; some other scholars concurred that the common causes of substance abuse among men include the following:

i. *Masculinity and self-medication*

Men are taught from early that men should take risks and do not display any signs of weakness. As a result of such gender-related expectations, men involve themselves in dangerous activities to prove their masculinity. This includes the use of drugs and substances. Furthermore, masculinity impacts the heath-seeking behavior of men for treatment of mental healthcare services as it may be regarded as a sign of being a coward and will put stain in their expectant masculinity [32, 33]. Masculine norms internalize help-seeking behavior [34]. Therefore, as a result, they self-medicate with drugs and substances. Most individuals with substance abuse exhibit signs and symptoms such as mood changes, anger, and sadness [26].

ii. *Pressure from life circumstances*

Stressful life events play a major role in substance abuse among men. A study conducted among American African men revealed that unintentional drug use and substance abuse inflicted mental illness. Social issues such as struggling to succeed at work and lack of support family members, and financial struggles were a trigger to substance use and abuse [35].

iii. *Grief and loss of a loved one*

Complicated grief is prolonged bereavement-specific disorder with substantial psychological and physical consequences. Individuals deal with complicated grief differently. More complicated grief represents a greater risk of substance misuse and abuse [36]. Substance abuse has become a coping method to avoid dealing painful experiences such as grief and significant loss among men. Loss of a loved one is tied to emotions strains and poses suicidal ideation among individuals [37].

iv. *Trauma and negative childhood experiences*

Substance abuse and posttraumatic stress disorders are comorbid. Due to exposure of the traumatic events, individuals self-medicate with drugs and alcohol to deal with anxiety, subsequently leading to substance abuse [38].

5.2 Domestic violence as a coping mechanism

Domestic violence has been gradually increasing worldwide; it is associated with the gender role inequalities such as abusing women as an exertion of power and assuming the traditional masculine role [39, 40]. However, despite the gender role inequalities as an expression of masculinities, domestic violence could be a result of substance abuse by perpetrators and could also be associated as a mechanism to deal with internal conflicts and mental health problems among men. The World Health Organization affirmed that as a result of societal expectations and traditional masculinities discouraging men from seeking help, instead they lash out and abuse their families as a coping mechanism to deal with the mental health problems. Although there is limited literature pertinent to domestic violence as a coping mechanism, majority of studies focus on the impact of abuse on the mental health of both men and women. Therefore, this requires further studies looking more into association of domestic abuse by men and their mental health status during the abuse toward their families.

5.3 Informal support

Dealing with mental health-sensitive issues among men is a difficult issue due to poor health-seeking behavior. Men often seek informal support from non-health professionals, and this includes family and friends; sometimes, they do not seek any support at all. They rather deal with such issues alone [40].

6. Cultural norms as a major barrier to seeking mental health services

Men are more disinclined to seek help with regard to health problems than women; this has mostly been associated with traditional ideas of masculinity [34]. Men are burdened by what is expected of them, and the masculinity roles are expected to assume in their lives. As a result, many young men are soldiering on nonetheless and swallow their own feelings, and this comes to a point the men reach a stage to take own life. While men are trying to accomplish the societal respects as a consequence of higher expectations from them, their stress levels increase and their mental health mostly remains unchecked (**Figure 3**) [28].

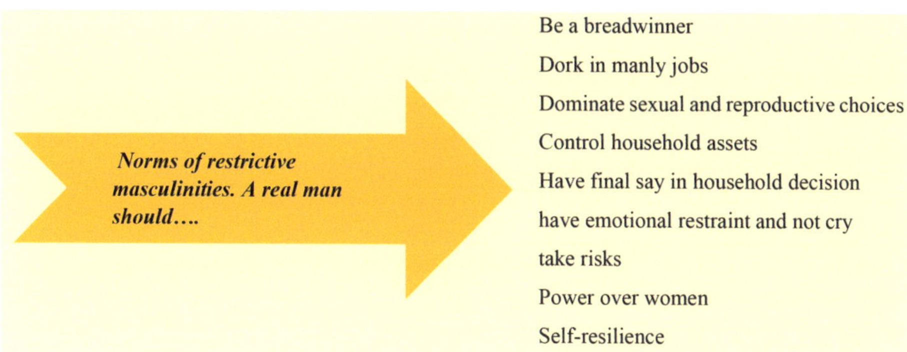

Figure 3.
Masculinity norms of what men are expected to be [41].

6.1 Theories of masculinity and its effects on men's mental health

Masculinity includes cultural and social norms, behaviors, and practices. The concept of toxic masculinity aims at underlining how certain socially constructed definition of masculinity can be detrimental to a society, men, and women [42]. The numerous reasons behind toxic masculinity include biological and social dimensions. The social dimensions include the family and friend's environment, educational system, workplace, and religion [43]. Examples of toxic masculinity include overtly aggression of a man to a female to show power and dominance and also never showing emotions as they are viewed as feminine trait because it shows weakness. Toxic masculinity affects and harms the one's mental health [44]. This may be one of the reasons why men commit suicide. A study conducted on social media, behavior, toxic masculinity, and depression revealed that toxic masculinity is associated with depression [45].

7. Strategies to improve access to men-centered mental healthcare services

7.1 Teamwork

One of the key aspects of this approach is the recognition that professionals should work as a team and that high-quality healthcare involves improving relationships between staff and between patients and their families [46].

7.2 An intervention aiming to reduce self-stigma associated with mental health problems

Reducing stigma associated with healthcare, ill-health, and health-seeking behaviors by addressing internalized stigma with men. Reducing healthcare worker stigma associated with healthcare, ill-health, and health-seeking behaviors by providing sensitization training for healthcare workers [5]. A male-sensitive brochure to address help-seeking in depressed men, an intervention aiming to reduce self-stigma associated with mental health problems [29].

7.3 Key processes that improved help-seeking attitudes, intentions, or behaviors for men

The use of role models to convey information, psychoeducational material to improve mental health knowledge, assistance with recognizing and managing symptoms, active problem-solving tasks, motivating behavior change, signposting services, and finally, content that built on positive male traits were important processes that improved help-seeking attitudes, intentions, or behaviors for men.

7.4 Public awareness campaigns and interventions designed to improve men's psychological help-seeking

These include campaign focusing on educating the public about depression in men. This awareness can be motivated through advertisements and campaigns such as the Real men Real Depression campaign with emphasis on targeting at-risk subgroups first and then the general community [28].

7.5 Psychological referral

When men seek help from mental health experts, men-centered therapy that emphasizes enhancing the client's capacity for accepting their circumstances is of important. A concise structured therapeutic plan that is clear and straightforward will be more effective and encourage client trust in both the therapist and the course of treatment [28].

7.6 Bias reduction

Every step of the therapy process should take the client's uniqueness and culture into account. In other words, prejudice reduction should be prioritized at all client contact levels. The client's belief that men cannot experience mental health issues could be a barrier to treatment acceptance and compromise the therapy's efficacy. Thus, taking into account this cultural idea will aid in neutralizing any potential therapeutic bias. According to the client's needs, it is suggested that the therapist take into account the numerous types of biases, including therapist, cultural, and individual [28].

7.7 Demand

A range of social and behavior change communication (SBCC) interventions are needed, including mass media communication, community outreach, and peer education. Such SBCC approaches need to provide clear, factual, and unbiased information, to increase men's knowledge and self-efficacy; promote communication among men, among peers, and within families; and encourage men to seek care and use services [5].

8. Policy considerations to men's mental health

8.1 Platform for men's mental health

Although there are mental health services available in South Africa, attention should be mostly directed toward creating more platforms to address sensitive issues affecting men, consequently leading to suicide. The extensive platforms should be of nonjudgmental and focused on self-determination as well as building the mental well-being of men. Studies revealed that men die of depression and substance abuse disorders; and these are mostly liked due to financial stress, pressure from society and family as well as cultural and social norms. Furthermore, to curve suicide mortalities globally, it is recommended that men's mental health should be given more attention and more research should be done in exploring strategies and procedures to address men's sensitive issues with the aim to reduce mortalities due to suicide among men. Therefore, health practitioners should be trained to have an effective role in asking men about their sensitive mental health issues to determine the root of the mental health problems [40]. Online support forums should be made available where men can vent their stories, experiences, and receive support [2]. In addition to addressing men's mental health issues, peer-led men-only groups may improve the self-esteem and confidence of men in disclosing weaknesses [34].

8.2 Mental health before cultural norms

Despite our pride toward our culture and religions, some of the cultural norms put an extensive pressure in men, leading them to most likely resort into depression and substance abuse, subsequently leading to suicide attempts. Traditional masculinities and cultural expectations for men's behaviors discourage men to recognize and seek mental healthcare services; consequently, these mental health problems remain hidden or manifest in disastrous ways such as domestic violence, substance abuse, and sometimes suicide [2]. Therefore, it is recommended that human lives should be a priority before our cultural norms. Putting the mental health needs of men before our cultural norms is most likely to save the lives of men worldwide. Moreover, healthcare professionals should be trained on the impact of masculine norms on the mental health [34].

9. Conclusion

Changes should be made on the existing social and cultural norms as they suppress the mental health being of men. To reduce the statistics of suicides mortalities due to mental distress, interventions should be implemented from early childhood stages to address gender variations. Despite the masculine advantages, men should not be raised different from women. This could reduce the implications of societal expectations and cultural norms in the mental being of men. Programs addressing the mental well-being of men should be vigorously implemented and inform men that there is no shame in seeking mental healthcare services and there is no shame in crying. This could possibly reduce completed suicides and suicide ideation among men as well as substance abuse and domestic violence.

Author details

Mxolisi Welcome Ngwenya and Gsakani Olivia Sumbane*
University of Limpopo, Polokwane, South Africa

*Address all correspondence to: gsakani.sumbane@ul.ac.za

References

[1] Galderisi S, Heinz A, Kastrup M, Beezhold J, Sartorius N. Toward a new definition of mental health. World Psychiatry. 2015;**14**(2):231

[2] World Health Organization. WHO global meeting to accelerate progress on SDG target 3.4 on noncommunicable diseases and mental health, 9-12 December 2019, Muscat, Oman: meeting report. 2020

[3] World Health Organization. Suicide Worldwide in 2019: Global Health Estimates. Geneva: World Health Organization; 2021. Licence: CC BY-NC-SA 3.0 IGO

[4] Mthembu ME. Factors affecting men's health care seeking behaviour and use of services: A case study of Inanda Township, Durban [Doctoral dissertation]. 2015

[5] (NDoH) National Department of Health South Africa. The South African National Integrated Men's Health Strategy 2020-2025. Pretoria, SA; December 2020

[6] Brådvik L. Suicide risk and mental disorders. International Journal of Environmental Research and Public Health. 2018;**15**(9):2028

[7] Schumacher H. Why More Men than Women Die by Suicide. London: BBC Future; 2019. Available from: https://www.bbc.com/future/article/20190313-why-more-men-kill-themselves-than-women

[8] Available from: https://www.bing.com/ck/a?!&&p=708264092b2acd81JmltdHM9MTY2NDE1MDQwMCZpZ3VpZD0yYzBmMDliOS01OTlkLTY1YTEtMDU2YS0wNjFlNTgxNzY0NjgmaW5zaWQ9NTEyMg&ptn=3&hsh=3&fclid=2c0f09b9-599d-65a1-056a-061e58176468&u=a1aHR0cHM6Ly93d3cuY2RjLmdvdi9zdWljaWRlL2ZhY3RzL2luZGV4Lmh0bWw&ntb=1 accessed September 2022

[9] Available from: https://afsp.org/suicide-statistics/ accessed September 2022

[10] Henriksson M, Wall A, Nyberg J, Adiels M, Lundin K, Bergh Y, et al. Effects of exercise on symptoms of anxiety in primary care patients: A randomized controlled trial. Journal of Affective Disorders. 2022;**297**:26-34

[11] Yu R, Chen Y, Li L, Chen J, Guo Y, Bian Z, et al. Factors associated with suicide risk among Chinese adults: A prospective cohort study of 0.5 million individuals. PLoS Medicine. 2021;**18**(3):e1003545

[12] Jang H, Lee W, Kim YO, Kim H. Suicide rate and social environment characteristics in South Korea: The roles of socioeconomic, demographic, urbanicity, general health behaviors, and other environmental factors on suicide rate. BMC Public Health. 2022;**22**(1):1-10

[13] Kim KA, Kim YE, Yoon SJ. Descriptive epidemiology on the trends and sociodemographic risk factors of disease burden in years of life lost due to suicide in South Korea from 2000 to 2018. BMJ Open. 2021;**11**(2):e043662

[14] Statistics. Suicide rates by gender 2010-2021 in South Korea. Korea: state of mental health; 2021

[15] Mars B, Burrows S, Hjelmeland H, Gunnell D. Suicidal behaviour across the African continent: A review of the literature. BMC Public Health. 2014;**14**(1):1-14

[16] Govender RD, Schlebusch L. A suicide risk screening scale for HIV infected persons in the immediate postdiagnosis

period. Southern African Journal of HIV Medicine. 2013;**14**(2):58-63

[17] Kootbodien T, Naicker N, Wilson KS, Ramesar R, London L. Trends in suicide mortality in South Africa, 1997 to 2016. International Journal of Environmental Research and Public Health. 2020;**17**(6): 1850

[18] Meissner B, Bantjes J, Kagee A. I would rather just go through with it than be called a wussy: An exploration of how a group of young South African men think and talk about suicide. American Journal of Men's Health. 2016;**10**(4):338-348

[19] Affleck W, Carmichael V, Whitley R. Men's mental health: Social determinants and implications for services. The Canadian Journal of Psychiatry. 2018;**63**(9):581-589

[20] Kizza D, Knizek BL, Kinyanda E, Hjelmeland H. Men in despair: A qualitative psychological autopsy study of suicide in Northern Uganda. Transcultural Psychiatry. 2012;**49**(5):696-717

[21] Ogrodniczuk JS, Oliffe JL. Men and depression. Canadian Family Physician. 2011;**57**(2):153-155

[22] Ward E, Wiltshire JC, Detry MA, Brown RL. African American men and women's attitude toward mental illness, perceptions of stigma, and preferred coping behaviors. Nursing Research. 2013;**62**(3):185

[23] Swetlitz N. Depression's problem with Men. AMA Journal of Ethics. 2021;**23**(7):586-589

[24] McKenzie SK, Collings S, Jenkin G, River J. Masculinity, social connectedness, and mental health: Men's diverse patterns of practice. American Journal of Men's Health. 2018;**12**(5):1247-1261

[25] Oliffe JL, Ogrodniczuk JS, Bottorff JL, Johnson JL, Hoyak K. "You feel like you can't live anymore": Suicide from the perspectives of Canadian men who experience depression. Social Science & Medicine. 2012;**74**(4):506-514

[26] Townsend MC, Morgan KI. Psychiatric Mental Health Nursing: Concepts of Care In Evidence-Based Practice. Philadelphia PA: FA Davis; 2017

[27] Booysen D, Mahe-Poyo P, Grant R. The experiences and perceptions of mental health service provision at a primary health centre in the Eastern Cape. South African Journal of Psychiatry. 2021;**27**(1):1-8

[28] Ezeugwu CR, Ojedokun O. Masculine norms and mental health of African men: What can psychology do? Heliyon. 2020;**6**(12):e05650

[29] Sagar-Ouriaghli I, Godfrey E, Bridge L, Meade L, Brown JS. Improving mental health service utilization among men: A systematic review and synthesis of behavior change techniques within interventions targeting help-seeking. American Journal of Men's Health. 2019;**13**(3):1557988319857009

[30] American Psychiatric Association. Depressive Disorders: DSM-5® Selections. Arlington VA: American Psychiatric Pub; 2015

[31] Substance Abuse and Mental Health Services Administration. Key substance use and mental health indicators in the United States: Results from the 2020 National Survey on Drug Use and Health (HHS Publication No. PEP21-07-01-003, NSDUH Series H-56). Rockville, MD: Center for Behavioral Health Statistics and Quality, Substance Abuse and Mental Health Services Administration. 2021

[32] Lakin DP, Win KS, Aung H, Soe KNC, Kyi B, Marcell AV, et al. Masculinity and mental health treatment initiation for former political prisoners in Yangon,

Myanmar–A qualitative investigation. BMC Public Health. 2021;**21**(1):1-10

[33] Common Causes of Substance Use in Men — High Focus Centers. Available from: pyramidhealthcarepa.com) accessed September 2022

[34] Staiger T, Stiawa M, Mueller-Stierlin AS, Kilian R, Beschoner P, Gündel H, et al. Masculinity and help-seeking among men with depression: A qualitative study. Frontiers in Psychiatry. 2020;**11**:599039

[35] Maclean JC, Webber D, French MT. Workplace problems, mental health and substance use. Applied Economics. 2015;**47**(9):883-905

[36] Parisi A, Sharma A, Howard MO, Wilson AB. The relationship between substance misuse and complicated grief: A systematic review. Journal of Substance Abuse Treatment. 2019;**103**:43-57

[37] Woodford MS. Men, substance use, and grief. In: Grief Work in Addictions Counseling. New York: Routledge; 2022. pp. 86-98

[38] María-Ríos CE, Morrow JD. Mechanisms of shared vulnerability to post-traumatic stress disorder and substance use disorders. Frontiers in Behavioral Neuroscience. 2020;**14**:6

[39] Khan ME, Townsend JW, Pelto PJ, editors. Sexuality, gender roles and domestic violence in South Asia, New York: Population Council; 2014

[40] Morgan K, Williamson E, Hester M, Jones S, Feder G. Asking men about domestic violence and abuse in a family medicine context: Help seeking and views on the general practitioner role. Aggression and Violent Behavior. 2014;**19**(6):637-642

[41] Iwamoto DK, Gordon DM, Oliveros A, Perez-Cabello MA, Brabham T, Lanza AS, et al. The role of masculine norms and informal support on mental health in incarcerated men. Psychology of Men & Masculinity. 2012;**13**(3):283

[42] Rotundi L. The issue of toxic masculinity. [Bachelor's Thesis, LUISS Guido Carli]. 2020. LUISS Biblioteca. Available from: http://tesi.luiss.it/27362

[43] Gail S, Tessarek A. Social Frameworks International Business Management, 2021. Berlin: Berlin School of law and economics; 2020

[44] Grewal, A. The Impact of Toxic Masculinity On Men's Mental Health. Washington: University of Washington Tacoma, Sociology Student Work Collection. 2020;**68**

[45] Parent MC, Gobble TD, Rochlen A. Social media behavior, toxic masculinity, and depression. Psychology of Men & Masculinities. 2019;**20**(3):277

[46] Gask L, Coventry P. Person-centred mental health care: The challenge of implementation. Epidemiology and Psychiatric Sciences. 2012;**21**(2):139-144

Chapter 6

The 4H and 4T Pediatric Early Acute Support in the Deteriorating Child: Competent Staff Instead Experts Facing the New Threats, and New Approaches Can Reduce Mortality – Experience in Guatemala

Luis Augusto Moya-Barquín, Diana Leticia Coronel-Martínez and Robert Conrad Sierra Morales

Abstract

Pediatric advanced life support courses provide widespread education on recognizing and treating cardiac arrest in children. Their main goal is to teach the cardiopulmonary resuscitation (CPR) sequence and improve early recognition and treatment of leading causes for better survival rates. Initially, there were four "H" and four "T" conditions, but now 12 are recognized. The 12 reversible conditions, categorized as "H's" and "T's," consist of seven starting with "H" and five starting with "T." The "H's" include hypovolemia, hypoxia, hydrogen ion excess (acidosis), hypoglycemia, hypokalemia, hyperkalemia, and hypothermia. The "T's" include tension pneumothorax, tamponade—cardiac, toxins, thrombosis (pulmonary embolus), and thrombosis (myocardial infarction). Finding specific training for these conditions in structured courses can be challenging. However, understanding their physiological basis enables healthcare providers to detect and treat them early, leading to improved outcomes and reduced mortality rates in Guatemala. In response to the COVID-19 outbreak, a regular course on managing these conditions was initiated for pediatric intensivists, pediatricians, and healthcare staff. In 2022, the Continuing Medical Education program at Universidad de San Carlos de Guatemala extended coverage to 134 physicians in rural areas and 50 pediatric intensivists from the Sociedad Latinoamericana de Cuidado Intensivo Pediátrico (SLACIP).

Keywords: cardiopulmonary resuscitation, 4H & 4T, cardiac arrest, cardiopulmonary resuscitation education, cardiac arrest causes, reversible causes cardiac arrest

1. Introduction

The widespread education and goals of the pediatric advanced life support (PALS) have been demonstrated as an important competence that implies skills and attitudes related to decision-making and teamwork in the healthcare personnel. In high-income countries, when personnel is hired, this becomes a requirement for the startup and it is expected, as a hospital requirement, to keep and update certification [1–5].

PALS guidelines published by the American Heart Association (AHA) are designed for resuscitation in a broad range of scenarios and environments. In general, the main goal of several life support courses is to learn the sequence for cardiopulmonary resuscitation; the related algorithm for cardiac arrest evaluation always goes back to the recognition of its leading causes that need rapid assessment and treatment to increase survival. These conditions were initially described as 4 "H" and 4 "T" (H and T are related to the first letter of each of the conditions). Currently, several centers and healthcare providers recognize 12. The 12 H's and T's are reversible conditions, of these seven start with H and five start with T. These conditions are:

- H's: hypovolemia, hypoxia, hydrogen ion excess (acidosis), hypoglycemia, hypokalemia, hyperkalemia, and hypothermia.

- T's: tension pneumothorax, tamponade—cardiac, toxins, thrombosis (pulmonary embolus), and thrombosis (myocardial infarction).

It is not easy to find specific training for H & T's conditions in structured courses. Understanding the physiological basis of these conditions can give the healthcare provider the opportunity of an early detection and treatment of these life-threatening conditions.

The required competencies, the understanding, and the metacognition of these conditions need more expertise than "getting the pass score" in the PALS course.

In developing countries, the main barrier to taking the PALS courses is the copyright and the merchandise; this course has been registered as intellectual property implying a payment for using the license. Currently in developing countries, the deployment of basic biological and educational science in the training and performance of the residents is still the focus. The quality assurance knowledge and the adherence to guidelines, protocols, and procedures still require a cultural change and the development of the teamwork concept; this is not only about technology [4].

Even knowing that the basic life support and the advanced life support courses are designed for the early recognition and treatment of the imminent cardiac arrest, the availability in low- and middle-income countries is very limited due to the market implications and subsequent cost, without any consideration about the design or quality of the training during the course. The AHA (American Heart Association) courses are more extended with all the implications already described [1–5].

Since the 1990s, the cardiopulmonary resuscitation courses in collaboration with colleagues from the USA begun; it was yearly and primarily directed to people who can speak English. Some years, the course was discontinued, and during other years, it was taken by the exact same group due to the English language barrier and consequence never disseminated among others, losing a lot of good opportunities for distributing knowledge to healthcare professionals only due to language barrier that could be easily solved.

In 2003, at the Pediatric Intensive Care Unit in Hospital General San Juan de Dios, we started endorsing and implementing standard guidelines for pediatric traumatic brain injury and goal-directed therapy, using validated protocols, guidelines, and quality assurance in the formation of human resources and for clinical management. Between 1995 and 2003, a very high mortality rate in 12-bed wards in the national reference hospital in Guatemala was reported; the mean Pediatric Risk of Mortality score—PRISM III was 6–9 points in deceased patients.

In 2009, the RIBEPCI (Red Iberoamericana para el Estudio de la Parada Cardiorrespiratoria en la Infancia) started working with us in Guatemala; this group endorsed the Grupo Guatemalteco de Reanimación Avanzada Pediátrica (GRAP) GUATEMALA, who can keep in a local manner a regular structure and education of the Health Care Staff Spanish and with nonprofit purposes. This course gives the possibility to the healthcare providers of delivering these courses to their own staff once they are certified. The RIBEPCI courses are based on and endorsed by the European Resuscitation Council (ERC).

In 2009, the Postgraduate course of Pediatric Intensivists began with the endorsement of the Universidad de San Carlos de Guatemala.

The RIBEPCI experience and GRAP GUATEMALA experience in the Hospital General San Juan de Dios were combined and led to the creation of SOYUTZ Pediatric Emergencies Simulation Center in 2014. The word soyutz, it is a mixed word from Russian Soyuz that means "union" and Utz in quiche Mayan language that means "good" and the word soyutz means good union, this is representing teamwork).

There is an important need of retaining trained staff and of maintaining them updated, this will allow an integrated flow in the scope of an attention model based on decision-making process sharing for optimizing the time-sensitive interventions. The fragmentation of healthcare in several specialized medicine fields results very frequently in an orphan patients; these "orphan" patients are in the middle of several medical specialties and even with an overlapping attention, the decision-making is not shared and could become a great conflict. The artificially separated attention of patients who need noninterventional attention and the patients that could require a surgical intervention becomes a problem in facilities of developing countries; in this kind of setting, we can find a primary care physician able to solve several conditions; and the level of the University hospitals would be very important that surgery, orthopedics, trauma anesthesia, pediatrics, emergency, and pediatric intensive care residents share the algorithms for recognition and treatment, no matter if these belong to the pediatric field or to the primary care field [6].

The classical approach for diagnosing sepsis, trauma, burns, surgical conditions, pneumonia, dengue, hypovolemic shock caused by diarrhea, diabetic ketoacidosis, and even COVID-19, among others, using the construction of a concept adding signs and symptoms with some grade of sensibility and specificity, could lead to diagnostic criteria with a high level of uncertainty; this also generates important delays for patient stabilization in emergency departments and hospitalization wards. This situation plus, the decision-making about referring a patient to a healthcare facility without solving access barriers like distance and quality of the roads, constitute a model of delays avoiding a fast-track process of recognition–stabilization, increasing the negative impact of hypoxia, ischemia, and reperfusion injury [7–9].

Patients with trauma or requiring surgery, could also have a congenital condition or an oncologic diagnosis; these adaptative conditions related to the disease, their related treatment, and potential complications should be considered before the surgery due to their very high possible relationship with deterioration and cardiac arrest when these are underestimated. In the perioperative environment, most of the arrests are witnessed, the patients are being monitored at the time of arrest, and the reason for the arrest may be related to the intervention or treatment. In this chapter, the perioperative period is defined as the period in which the patient is cared for by the anesthesia team and focuses on events that occur in the operating room, procedural areas, and diagnostic imaging areas from the moment that the patient is seen for the first time by the anesthesia team until the patient is transferred to another service or is discharged to home or to another facility. Cardiac arrest is defined as a "no-flow" state requiring chest compressions (open or closed chest) or failure to wean from cardiopulmonary bypass.

The cardiac arrest is categorized as out-of-hospital cardiac arrest (OOHCA) or in-hospital cardiac arrest (IHCA), both requiring a structured attention, using good quality cardiopulmonary resuscitation; the issue with this is that both conditions imply a pulseless event or a life-threatening condition. The cardiac arrest has three phases, and these phases have important implications for therapeutic actions. The cardiopulmonary resuscitation utilizes a rhythm-based approach, and the problem is that this action only considers the time elapsed after the onset of cardiac arrest. The cardiac arrest is addressed using the three-phase time-dependent model. This model is clearly time-dependent considering for clinical evaluation "0 min" as the startup [10].

The three phases in this model are:

a. First phase (electrical): Begins with the onset of cardiac arrest and lasts for about 5 min; the therapeutic gold standard for this phase is early and rapid defibrillation.

b. Second phase (circulatory): Exists between 5 and 10 min after the initiation of arrhythmic cardiac arrest. The treatment objective in this phase should be the maximization of blood flow to the myocardium.

c. Third phase (metabolic): Begins 10 min after the initiation of cardiac arrest and is related in proportion to high mortality.

It is very important to understand that the underlying processes of cardiac arrest and the related physiological conditions could start several minutes before [10].

The overall goal of all perioperative resuscitative efforts or stabilization like the golden hour in medical conditions is to minimize this no-flow period and to maximize the chance of spontaneous circulation return. Whereas the indications for resuscitation outside of the operating room may be simple (loss of consciousness, loss of pulse, etc.), the indications in the perioperative period may be more complex. They may include inadequate heart rate or blood pressure based on age, inadequate minute ventilation, cyanosis, failure of noninvasive blood pressure monitoring or pulse oximetry, loss of arterial waveform, or a sudden change in the end-tidal carbon dioxide (ETCO2) waveform or value.

For understanding the physiological instability, it is necessary to understand how the body's dynamic balance is related to a predetermined range of values in healthy conditions, and the most common for age and gender (e.g., perfusion, level of consciousness, blood pressure, work of breathing, and metabolic state) with or without clinical intervention.

The approach to organ dysfunction or failure cannot be done when one or more vital organ dysfunction or failure is due to chronic adaptation, with or without severe impairment, dysfunction, or external support. In fact, the main cause of an imminent life-threatening condition is the unrecognized process of deterioration due to treatment failure and deficient monitoring with the addition of poor knowledge of any chronic adaption of the patient. High accuracy and low opportunity (HALO) are required for improving any time-sensitive intervention. The HALO applicability will require at the same time healthcare workers with enough skills and with strong commitment and knowledge for decision-making and execution of any needed action in all patients, requiring or not an intervention [11–15]. The early approach is based on the probability and uncertain odds of potential reversibility. The recognition is time-sensitive, and this could help a situation may be reversible with defined goals and objectives of directed management. Sometimes, the organ dysfunction may persist and develop to adaptative physiology in case leading to a condition that could be technology-dependence or chronic. Is there when Sir William Osler's quote describes the everyday practice of medicine "A science of uncertainty and an art of probability" [16].

There is a need for developing acute care in any place; the recognition and evaluation of the acute patient have common bases and could be done in any location outside the emergency department (ED) or the pediatric intensive care unit (PICU); sometimes could be related with surgical process (before operating room and recovery room). For making possible acute care independent of the location, teamwork has the most important role in recognizing, approaching, treating, and monitoring any pediatric patient.

It is important to recognize that the location sometimes is not designed and equipped with the optimal resources. The attention of the patient will be resource-availability independent. In the developing countries' settings, attention is based on the equipment and facilities that are more focused on diagnostic or laboratory resources with a lot of delays, omissions, and pitfalls in attention [17–19].

The education process from basic concepts and its evolution is needed for allowing the growth of the healthcare worker in autonomy and responsibility. This process is a shared pathway that needs the supervision of a mentor; at some point, new mentors will be formed, able to train and able to work and educate as peers. In this moment, the student reaches the finest level of competence: the leadership. In the everyday teamworking process, the importance of the followership is growing; this very important and special skill is based in the capability of putting aside ego, seniority, and hierarchy for promoting the empowerment from the rest of the team. The

Level	Novice	Advanced	Competent	Competent advanced	Expert
Miller's pyramid	Know	Know how	Show how	Do	Teach others
Bloom's taxonomy	Remember enlist	Explain interpret	Apply solve	Predict criticize	Planify design
Challenges			+	+++	++++
Cultural competencies		+	+++	++++	+++
Esencial competencies	+	+++	++++	+++	++
Skills	+++	++++	+++	++	
Knowledge	++++	+++	++		

Table 1.
Education matrix for learning process.

competence model based on the Dunning–Kruger effect promotes self-confidence by using the capability to respond with responsibility. Based on Miller's Pyramid, Bloom's Taxonomy, and the International Pediatric Simulation Society, we can build an education matrix for learning process presented in **Table 1**.

2. Academic content

2.1 Dominion level

It is necessary to understand, in the education settings for medical students, nurses, and residents, how to have more operative performance to deploy anywhere the capabilities and response. The impact of the trained freshmen physicians is based on the opportunity to do appropriate and opportune interventions, the use of the resources, the proportionality of care, and the monitoring and treatment interventions.

It is different to define the sailing course and the destination of navigation, in this part, it is important to define routes and could be important to understand the steps and the sequence and the consequences of each step in order to teach the approach. The SODOTO methodology (See One, Do One, Teach One) for teaching and learning skills not necessarily is accurate when we review the cumulative sum analysis of the learning curve, based on patient safety. The cumulative supervised task requires enough amount for receiving the feedback and promoting the feedforward for making with reduced error any procedure or decision-making process. The experience of the 10,000 hours to reach mastery and the assessment using risk matrices is focused on the practice time using the most frequent scenarios in daily practice and the evaluation of the consequences of different decisions and their impact.

In PICU setting, is very important to know, to teach, to audit, to improve, and to learn step by step any process. A sequence of steps using mandatory commands (written process with sequences in programming imperative commands START, IF THEN, YES, NO, AND, OR FINISH) instead of flowcharts that could be confusing, the addition of the critical path method to distribute tasks and the crew resource management methodology for distributing the workload are the rules. All these allow the staff to track all the processes. The importance of having the algorithms using commands and tracked standard operative procedures (SOPs) is a blueprint for educative and performance purposes [20–22].

Nowadays is very frequent to find in our ward complex patients or technology dependent, medical education is based on diagnosis, syndromes, and diseases but not on ongoing processes and the tag to define one of those is not clear in the adaptative balance of the patient in these conditions.

It is very important to speed the early recognition of the signs of deterioration instead of being worried about the speed of the appearance of the signs of deterioration; this is the reason why monitoring is the basic recognition tool of a patient in a deteriorating process, with an apparent acute or sudden onset of illness in the settings of the compensated or decompensated shock, respiratory arrest, and cardiopulmonary arrest. Patients with chronic conditions who develop acute critical illness/deterioration needs more close monitoring. This may include patients with chronic conditions (e.g., cerebral palsy, chronic renal disease, etc.) who develop acute critical illness when the basic start is not necessarily healthy.

Potential reversibility is a very common attribute of critical illness in pediatric patients with suspected, probable, or at risk of critical illness; they may have one or more abnormal physiological parameters or vital signs compared to healthy children.

The evaluation of the deteriorating process instead of the cut-point of failure, or the diagnosis itself of disease is more important. In pediatric patients, trying to define the persistence of a condition for more than 60 min (1 h) based on the physiological parameters or vital signs, that are references from previous healthy children like >95th or < 5th percentile, or > 2 or < 2 SD for age and gender, could be risky when the monitoring and the consecutive evaluations are hourly. The changes of the trends of the vital signs are very important for recognizing the acute deterioration and could be necessary to have reevaluations at least every 15 min.

Qualitative and clinical physiological parameters or vital signs may include the pediatric assessment triangle and/or any pediatric early warning score or scale to promote early recognition and subsequent interventions. The used signs are mentioned in the following findings:

Central nervous system: Level of consciousness and response to external stimulus (awake, verbal response, pain response, or unresponsiveness) AVPU/Glasgow Coma Scale, pupils' size/reactivity-fixed, asymmetry.

Respiratory: Clinically, the breathing needs to be wide (lung expansion), correct (inflate in inspiration, deflate in expiration), and depth (enough volume and flow to expand the thorax). Signs of airway obstruction and respiratory distress, respiratory rate and effort, and the work of breath related to the respiratory pattern or mental status. Oxygen saturation is a measure to move the subjective evaluation of cyanosis.

Cardiovascular: Heart rate, systolic blood pressure, shock index (heart rate/ systolic blood pressure; normal value considered <1), capillary refill time, quality of central/ peripheral pulses, skin (temperature/color/perfusion), urine output, etc.

Nutritional problems could affect the clinical interpretation as in the case of core temperature, hepatomegaly, and signs of dehydration (e.g., sunken eyes, tears, dry mucosa), several studies report the bias in the accurate interpretation and pitfalls in the treatment of malnourished patients.

In terms of education, it is very important to share the decision-making process. The training should go from basic knowledge concepts to metacognition in explicit knowledge.

Human-dependent assessment can include but is not limited to vital signs, and the human-dependent monitoring/assessment needs an educational approach. The experience of COVID-19 in campaign hospitals demonstrated the urgency of competent staff instead of some experts.

The workload of the human-dependent assessment and monitoring of acute, critical, chronic, technology-dependent patients, requires a great number of hours/ shift but the pathway to reach and expert level is not always possible due to the high demands.

The approach of a suspected versus a confirmed diagnosis is quite different, in this case, the cut-point or the sum of the criteria sometimes could delay the treatment; other times, the syndromic approach could be useful for the recognition of patterns; this kind of pattern recognition is the base used for algorithms development, including artificial intelligence.

In statistics, likelihood is not the same as probability; we are performing for taking decisions in high uncertain, dynamic, and complex clinical scenarios with the addition of the technology and the devices that sustain a chronic patient. At this point, we need to teach critical thinking and the pattern recognition first and in a second step, make sure to teach also the adaptative physiology related to the medical device plus the function and programming of the medical device itself, including noninvasive or invasive mechanical ventilation. This technology is also related to resources for follow-up monitoring like X-rays, arterial blood gases, oximetry, end-tidal CO2, and others.

Pediatric patients with suspected, probable, deteriorating, or with critical illness may need frequent clinical evaluation and decision-making about the different trends or changes in patients' patterns. It is more important time-sensitive hands-on interventions instead of repetitive obtention of laboratory or diagnostic test. Those activities could be directed to the therapeutic interventions not only mobilization, suctioning, review of the tube's fixations, mouth care, repositioning, tracheostomy care, cold sponge bathing for fever, cleaning and dressing wounds/burns, or close follow,up of the fluids balance.

There is also a special group of patients who are in deterioration or at high risk related to traumatic or surgical conditions.

The priority in recognition is focused on pediatric patients with suspected, probable, or high risk for deterioration and evidence of critical illness; they may need time-sensitive life-supporting intervention, based on objectives and goals.

3. Children with comorbidities or preexisting conditions

The survival of patients from the Neonatal Intensive Care Unit (NICU), with congenital surgical or medical conditions is improving in developing countries. For this, recognition of co-morbidities and high-risk conditions is crucial.

In the PICU, the recognition of the risk of deterioration and/or exacerbation of any condition, or changes in the adaptative physiology is very important. Added malnutrition, obesity or overweight, congenital heart disease, oncologic diseases, primary immunosuppression or acquired immunosuppression like HIV/AIDS, transplant patients among others could increase the mortality rate in these patients.

Another important factors are the chronic pathologies with neurological disability, like cerebral palsy or neural tube defects and the use or dependence of invasive devices like shunt. These conditions imply adaptation of the patient's physiology. In these cases, the information given by the caregiver is fundamental for understanding the real changes of the mental status and behavior of the patient.

4. Essential and optimal resources for educational competencies and performance

Many times, the governance bodies believe that the growth in infrastructure and the recruitment of freshmen doctors are the solutions to the healthcare system; it is very common to think that hierarchy will give a person "magically," the required competencies, experience, and level of responsibility.

The definition of "Medical Attention Quality" will imply structure, process, and outcome. Any improvement of technology needs to be based on the comprehensive understanding of any tool as a resource (drug, device, laboratory test, X-ray, CT scan, among others) and is mandatory to understand any connected point as a chain of decision and iterative evaluations.

The physiology is the same in developing and developed countries, but to be effective, efficient, and explicit it is mandatory to be familiar with the local resources not only in the context of the access to some drugs (i.e., Amiodarone in several countries is substituted by Lidocaine, but Aminophylline is also widespread in some countries instead intravenous salbutamol and phenytoin used instead phosphenytoin). This is why we need to understand the reality of the environment where the educational process is being developed; in a first-level setting with fewer available resources, it could be more relevant to teach early noninvasive ventilation and bag-mask oxygenation instead of endotracheal intubation.

The essential resources that are known to be required in the health facilities besides the knowledge to solve medical problems and interventions including monitoring are enlisted but not reduced in the list below:

Central nervous system: Rewarming/cooling (targeting normothermia or therapeutic hypothermia), antidotes (naloxone and in the rural places consider acute or subacute organophosphates poisoning), first- and second-line antiepileptics, hyperosmolar therapy (mannitol/hypertonic saline), cerebrospinal fluid drainage or shunt for raised intracranial cerebral pressure (ICP), decompressive surgery, etc.

Respiratory: Continuous nebulizers, noninvasive/invasive ventilatory support from the high-flow nasal cannula (HFNC), bilevel positive airway pressure (BI-PAP), continuous positive airway pressure (CPAP) to the intubation drugs and supplies and mechanical ventilation as minimum, and thoracostomy tube.

Cardiovascular: Vascular access, intraosseous access, crystalloids, colloids, inotropes, vasopressors, vasodilators, cardiopulmonary resuscitation, pericardiocentesis, and blood products.

Metabolic: Feeding tubes, dextrose, bicarbonate, sodium, potassium, calcium, phosphorus, magnesium, and insulin.

Additional thrombolytics, heparin, and the supplies to make invasive procedures, and personal protective equipment for the health personnel.

5. Conclusions

Since 2003, the implemented educational process at the PICU in the Hospital San Juan de Dios in Guatemala showed a clear improvement in the medical attention and very clear impact on the mortality rate reduction. It is important to highlight that, during these years (from 2003 until now), we kept experiencing several economic constraints. Even with some improvements in equipment and resources, the major reason for the improvement has been the educational activities directed to the human resources at PICU.

On 2003, with a 12-bed PICU facility, 620 admissions per year were registered with 165 deaths; on 2022, with a 49-bed PICU, 99 deaths were reported. Currently, even the patients with the worst prognostic (average PRISM III score of 27 in 2022 compared to the average score of 9 in 2003) have better chances of survival. The 2019 COVID-19 pandemic gave us the opportunity of improving the on-site training and the virtual education using videos, simulation, remote training, and other resources.

Another important aspect during the pandemic was to increase the empathy for attending family and parents' needs. Situations like restricted access and the curfew among other conditions related to the pandemic were faced using different strategies like "phone access" and special support in cases of withholding and withdrawing treatment when parents were away and not easy to reach (i.e., living in remote areas).

After the COVID-19 pandemic in 2020, we started a regular course for teaching the management of H & T's for the pediatric intensivists, the pediatricians and the physicians, or health staff who need to be aware about the recognition and treatment of H & T's. In 2022, 134 physicians located in rural healthcare facilities were enrolled, the specialties of these physicians are anesthesiology, surgery, orthopedics, emergency care, and pediatrics, nurses were included. At the level of the Latino American Society of Pediatric Critical Care (Sociedad Latinoamericana de Cuidado Intensivo Pediátrico, SLACIP), 50 pediatric intensive care physicians were trained. This training now has the endorsement of the Continued Medical Education Department of the Universidad de San Carlos de Guatemala.

We believe that, worldwide, it is not only about improving the infrastructure, and the equipment, or purchasing new technology, or hiring more personnel; all these for sure are very valuable strategies; but also without education, none of this will work.

We need well-trained healthcare personnel; the key to this always will be education; we need to educate for improving the performance and the decision-making process; we need to track the improvement of the team. Negotiation, decision-making process, and teamwork are fundamental skills under the concept of command incidents system, knowing this, we could add another H and another T: Humanization and Teamwork.

Acknowledgements

We are thankful for the contribution of Jesús López-Herce MD, MSc, Raffo Escalante-Kanashiro MD, MSc, Hugo Loayza MD Msc, Carlos Román-Ramos MD, MSc and Manuel Correa, MD Msc. in the development of this approach and diffusion of the related knowledge.

Author details

Luis Augusto Moya-Barquín[1*], Diana Leticia Coronel-Martínez[2] and Robert Conrad Sierra Morales[1]

1 Pediatric Intensive Care Unit, Hospital General San Juan de Dios, Universidad de San Carlos de Guatemala, Guatemala City, Guatemala

2 Grupo de Reanimación Avanzada, Pediátrica—GRAP México, México City, México

*Address all correspondence to: sistemaluismoya@gmail.com

References

[1] Grzeskowiak M. The knowledge of the potential reversible causes (4H, 4T) in cardiac arrest and applying them while performing a successful resuscitation—a comparative study. Anestezjiologia I Ratownictwo. 2011;**5**:23-27

[2] Reddy DRS, Hanmandlu A. The 4 H's and T's: How reliable is this mnemonic in classifying etiologies of in-hospital cardiac arrests? Resuscitation. 2022;**175**:3-5. DOI: 10.1016/j.resuscitation.2022.03.035

[3] Monsieurs KG, Nolan JP, Bossaert LL, Greif R, Maconochie IK, Nikolaou NI, et al. European Resuscitation Council Guidelines for Resuscitation 2015: Section 1. Executive summary. Resuscitation. Oct 2015;**95**:1-80. DOI: 10.1016/j.resuscitation.2015.07.038. Epub 2015 Oct 15. PMID: 26477410

[4] Van den Bempt S, Wauters L, Dewolf P. Pulseless electrical activity: Detection of underlying causes in a prehospital setting. Medical Principles and Practice. 2021;**30**(3):212-222. DOI: 10.1159/000513431

[5] Jentzer JC, Clements CM, Wright RS, White RD, Jaffe AS. Improving survival from cardiac arrest: A review of contemporary practice and challenges. Annals of Emergency Medicine. 2016;**68**(6):678-689. DOI: 10.1016/j.annemergmed.2016.05.022

[6] Moya-Barquin LA. When "first do not harm" is not enough; guiding learning curve performance from novice to expert in pediatrics residents in Guatemala to reduce mortality. EC Paediatrics. 2019;**8**(7):566-573

[7] Moya-Barquin LA, Coronel-Martinez DL. Is not only to recognize "errare humanum est" (to err is human), instead we must promote for patient safety "meliorare humanum est, supra collaboratio maximi momenti" (improve is human, better working as a team). EC Paediatrics. 2019;**8**(10):1131-1136

[8] Moya-Barquin LA, Coronel-Martinez DL. In pandemic Covid-19 outbreak, we learned from the statement of Jfk to the George Floyd Claim; all inhabit this small planet, we are all mortal and... we can't breathe. EC Paediatrics. 2020;**9**(8):87-92

[9] Bukhari H, Andreatta P, Goldiez B, Rabelo L. A framework for determining the return on investment of simulation-based training in health care. Inquiry: A Journal of Medical Care Organization, Provision, and Financing. 2017;**54**:46958016687176. DOI: 10.1177/0046958016687176

[10] Wollocko BM, Papian-Gorji B, Yen W, Zahid U, Shah N, Steier K, et al. An overview of therapy guidelines for cardiac arrest and the potential benefits of hemoglobin-based oxygen carriers. Cardiogenetics. 2022;**12**:37-48. DOI: 10.3390/cardiogenetics12010004

[11] Nguyen HB, Daniel-Underwood L, Van Ginkel C, et al. An educational course including medical simulation for early goal-directed therapy and the severe sepsis resuscitation bundle: An evaluation for medical student training. Resuscitation. 2009;**80**(6):674-679. DOI: 10.1016/j.resuscitation.2009.02.021

[12] Choy CL, Liaw SY, Goh EL, See KC, Chua WL. Impact of sepsis education for healthcare professionals and students on learning and patient outcomes: A systematic review. The Journal of Hospital Infection. 2022;**122**:84-95. DOI: 10.1016/j.jhin.2022.01.004

[13] Talkhan H, Stewart D, McIntosh T, et al. Investigating clinicians' determinants of antimicrobial prescribing behaviour using the theoretical domains framework. The Journal of Hospital Infection. 2022;**122**:72-83. DOI: 10.1016/j.jhin.2022.01.007

[14] Trovato G. SEPSIS. Educational and best practice frontiers. Beyond the boundaries of fatality, enhancing clinical skills and precision medicine. Therapeutics and Clinical Risk Management. 2020;**16**:87-93. DOI: 10.2147/tcrm.s232530

[15] Payot C, Fehlmann CA, Suppan L, et al. Factors influencing physician decision making to attempt advanced resuscitation in asystolic out-of-hospital cardiac arrest. International Journal of Environmental Research and Public Health. 2021;**18**(16):8323. DOI: 10.3390/ijerph18168323

[16] Borghi L. William Osler, Medical history and the origins of the International Society for the History of Medicine. Vesalius. 2018;**24**:5-17. ISSN 1373-4857

[17] Cheng A, Nadkarni VM, Mancini MB, et al. Resuscitation education science: Educational strategies to improve outcomes from cardiac arrest: A scientific statement from the American Heart Association. Circulation. 2018;**138**(6):e82-e122. DOI: 10.1161/cir.0000000000000583

[18] Lambert V, Matthews A, MacDonell R, Fitzsimons J. Paediatric early warning systems for detecting and responding to clinical deterioration in children: A systematic review. BMJ Open. 2017;**7**(3):e014497. DOI: 10.1136/bmjopen-2016-014497

[19] Almblad AC, Målqvist M, Engvall G. From skepticism to assurance and control; implementation of a patient safety system at a pediatric hospital in Sweden. PLoS One. 2018;**13**(11):e0207744. DOI: 10.1371/journal.pone.0207744

[20] Kotsis SV, Chung KC. Application of the "see one, do one, teach one" concept in surgical training. Plastic and Reconstructive Surgery. 2013;**131**(5):1194-1201. DOI: 10.1097/PRS.0b013e318287a0b3

[21] Hirschl RB. The making of a surgeon: 10,000 hours? Journal of Pediatric Surgery. 2015;**50**(5):699-706. DOI: 10.1016/j.jpedsurg.2015.02.061

[22] Vatanpour S, Hrudey SE, Dinu I. Can public health risk assessment using risk matrices be misleading? International Journal of Environmental Research and Public Health. 2015;**12**(8):9575-9588. DOI: 10.3390/ijerph120809575

Section 3

Barriers and Opportunities to Access to Health Care and Universal Health Coverage

Chapter 7

The Road to Universal Coverage by the End of 2022, the Moroccan Challenge

Chakib Boukhalfa

Abstract

In the midst of a pandemic, Morocco is generalizing its social protection by 2025 and above all its health coverage by the end of this year, by enrolling 22 million beneficiaries in health insurance. How will a health system, already marked by numerous failures, be able to absorb 22 million new beneficiaries in order to reach 100% medical coverage of the Moroccan population by the end of this year? This is a commendable project, but it risks being a missed opportunity if we do not change the paradigm, governance, and organization of the Moroccan health system upstream in order to make it more efficient and more equitable. What are the obstacles and difficulties encountered by the health system, and what are the accompanying measures undertaken to accompany the overhaul of the Moroccan health system?

Keywords: health system, universal coverage, health insurance, overhaul of the health system, health financing

1. Introduction

Morocco is a country where public and private health care coexist. Similarly, in terms of financing, it is a multiple system that includes a basic compulsory health insurance scheme and mutual insurance companies and private insurance companies that provide basic and/or supplementary medical cover.

The Moroccan health system is confronted with a multitude of problems linked essentially to the double demographic and health transition, to the insufficiency of the sector's resources, and to the inequity in the financing of care.

In order to overcome these dysfunctions and improve the health of the population and ensure equality of access to care, the public authorities have embarked on a huge reform project concerning medical coverage and health financing.

The financing of the health system in the different countries of the world can be classified into two groups:

In most high-income countries, the health financing system provides universal health care coverage, whether through taxes or through social health insurance, thus avoiding households having to pay for care out of their own pockets when they need it, called a prepayment system.

In poor countries, with limited government resources, households often contribute directly to health financing by paying for care when and where it is received, known as a user-paid provider fee system, with the great risk of committing the population to catastrophic expenses.

The consequences of these can be devastating, as they can lead to massive debt, loss of assets, sale of essential assets, and even a spiral of poverty. To mitigate this risk, many countries are establishing social security, universal health insurance, or financial aid systems to help low-income people access health care without incurring catastrophic expenses. The development of equitable financing systems is therefore essential to improve access to health care and protect the poor from the catastrophic costs caused by poor health. It is therefore necessary to find effective social protection strategies, favoring risk pooling and prepayment systems, and not direct payment by the patient of health care providers which discourages the poor from using their services [1].

The level of overall health expenditure in Morocco is low and unit prices are high. Since 1997-1998, several efforts have been made to improve health financing in Morocco. However, the structure of financing has changed only slightly. Households still remain the main financer of health with a share of 45.6%, a drop of 5.1 points compared to the 2013 national health accounts [2]. This significant drop is explained, on the one hand, by the extension of medical coverage and, on the other hand, by the expansion of the list of reimbursable drugs, the promotion of generic drug prescriptions, and also the reduction in drug prices since 2014.

According to the latest national health accounts for 2018, collective and solidarity financing reached 53.3% in 2018 [2], exceeding 50% for the first time, compared to 46.8% in 2013. The improvement in solidarity financing constitutes a positive trend toward financial protection for the population, especially the most vulnerable groups.

However, despite this decline in out-of-pocket payments by households, the level recorded is still high by international standards.

To ensure equity and equality in the field of health, there is a fundamental step that a country can take, which is to move toward universal coverage. This means providing the population with social protection that allows them to have universal access to all the services they need. Whether universal coverage is financed by taxation, organized on the basis of a social insurance system, or both, the principles are the same: pooling of contributions paid in advance and using these funds to ensure accessible benefits and quality care for those who need it without exposing them to catastrophic costs.

Morocco has started the reform of health financing by adopting law n° 65–00 on the code of basic medical coverage with two schemes whose objective is to consolidate and converge all actions toward the common goal of universal health coverage. The aim is to consolidate and converge all actions toward the common objective of universal health coverage, thus ensuring equality and equity in access to care for the entire population without causing financial difficulties for users.

The first of the two schemes is a compulsory health insurance scheme for public sector employees and private sector employees, based on the principles and techniques of social insurance for the benefit of gainfully employed persons and pensioners. The second is a medical assistance scheme for the economically deprived, based on the principles of social assistance and national solidarity for the benefit of the deprived population.

The aim is to provide universal health care coverage, either through taxes or through social health insurance, so that households do not have to pay out of pocket for care when they need it.

The current organization of the Moroccan health system has several difficulties preventing the smooth progress toward universal coverage that need to be addressed to ensure equitable access and treatment for all people. What then are the obstacles and difficulties encountered by the health system, and what are the accompanying measures undertaken to accompany the redesign of the Moroccan health system?

2. Are we talking about a recast and not a reform

The royal speech of His Majesty Mohamed VI in 2018 had raised two points: The first is the rectification of the anomalies that mar the implementation of the health coverage program for the economically deprived, and the second is the in-depth overhaul of the national health system characterized by glaring inequalities and poor management.

Before talking about the path toward the achievement of universal coverage and the overhaul of the health system in the context of this achievement, we must recall an ideal health system. The health system is the set of human, material, and financial resources, institutions and activities designed to ensure the promotion, protection, restoration, and rehabilitation of the health of the population. Financial activities go beyond health care (inpatient and outpatient) and medical goods to other health-related sectors, namely education, hygiene, community health prevention, and research.

Such a system must first of all be comprehensive, allowing for a global care of users with curative but also, and above all, preventive care, rehabilitation, and health promotion. Secondly, it must be geographically and economically accessible, that is, closer to the patient, and cost must not be an obstacle. Third, it must be technically and economically efficient. Fourth, it must be acceptable to the population with legitimate expectations. Fifth, it must be measurable and assessable, that is, easy to predict and measure via health indicators. Finally, it must be flexible and modifiable, with the capacity to adapt quickly in the event of the emergence of new needs. We have seen the vulnerability of health systems around the world. The most telling example is the Italian system, which has almost collapsed under the flow of patients. It has shown its inability to provide intensive care or resuscitation for all patients, forcing them into painful and difficult choices. All health systems around the world were overwhelmed by a common problem: They were unprepared and not resilient enough to cope with a massive influx of patients in a pandemic context.

Numerous reforms have been undertaken over the years, and several advances have been recorded, such as the vaccination program, mother and child health, the surveillance of communicable diseases, the eradication of certain diseases, free childbirth, and even the addition of an additional subsidy to public hospitals to compensate for the shortfall in hospital revenue, among others.

At the same time, Morocco has been on the road to universal health coverage since 2002 with the adoption of law n°65–00 on the Basic Medical Coverage (BMC) code. The first scheme implemented in 2005 was the Compulsory Health Insurance (CHI) for employees and pensioners in both the public and private sectors.

Subsequently, the basic medical coverage project continued with the launch of the pilot experiment in 2008 and the generalization in 2012 of the Medical Assistance Scheme (RAMED) for the benefit of the underprivileged population, followed by the entry into force of the compulsory health insurance for students in 2016, the adoption of the law relating to the compulsory health insurance for non-salaried workers in 2018, and the gradual publication of its implementing decrees (**Table 1**).

Population	Distribution
Population: National Fund for Social Welfare Organizations	8.8%
Population: National Health Insurance Fund	21.01%
Students: National Fund for Social Welfare Organizations	0.7%
Medical Assistance Scheme	30.5%
Population 114	4.4%
Royal Armed Forces Mutual Fund, Former Resistance fighters and others	4.6%
Total population coverage	**70.2%**

Source: Department of Planning and Financial Resources, compiled by the author.

Table 1.
Distribution of the Moroccan population covered according to the mode of coverage.

National Fund for Social Welfare Organizations (10%)	National Health Insurance Fund (90%)
• Public 3.20 million	• Private 7.6 million
• Population 114 0.26 million	• Population 114 1.3 million
• Students 0.23 million	• Non-salaried workers 11 million
	• Medical Assistance Scheme 11 million

Source: Department of Planning and Financial Resources, **completed by the author.**

Table 2.
Breakdown of the Moroccan population according to health insurance funds.

This process, crowned by the adoption of the framework law n° 09–21 relating to social protection, has made it possible to increase the rate of basic medical coverage of the Moroccan population from 16% in 2005 to 70.2% in 2020, that is, 25.2 million beneficiaries (all schemes combined), of which 11.17 million are the compulsory health insurance beneficiaries and 11 million are the Medical Assistance Scheme beneficiaries [3]. The goal is to reach 100% of the Moroccan population, through the integration of 11 million self-employed workers and 11 million current Assistance Scheme beneficiaries who will switch to compulsory health insurance (a total of 22 million citizens), before the end of 2022. They will have insurance covering the costs of treatment and hospitalization. The new distribution of the Moroccan population according to insurance bodies will be presented as depicted in **Table 2**.

Moreover, despite the efforts made, citizens continue to suffer from the many limitations of the current national health system. This transition has not prevented deep social and territorial divides from widening. It is true that the results of the National Population and Family Health Survey in 2018 revealed a significant reduction in the maternal mortality ratio, which fell to 72.6 maternal deaths per 100,000 live births from 112 in 2010, a reduction of 35%, and a reduction in the neonatal mortality rate, which fell from 21.7% per 1000 live births in 2010 to 13.6% in 2018, a reduction of 37%. Nevertheless, these results remain fragile as there are still remarkable differences between the data related to residence and welfare quintiles, hiding inequalities and inequities between groups of people and territories: The maternal mortality ratio is 44.6 deaths/100,000 newborns in urban areas and 111.1 deaths/100,000 newborns in rural areas [4].

3. Challenges to the Moroccan health system

To give an idea of the challenges to be met, Morocco has been ranked by the United Nations at the 110th place in terms of health system performance and 111th place in terms of equity.

The results of the Medical Assistance Scheme for the benefit of the underprivileged population, which was generalized in 2012, have not lived up to expectations, with delays in diagnosis and consultation appointments.

Almost a quarter of RAMED card patients who were supposed to receive free public health care are turning to private health care, with the risk of falling below the poverty line due to catastrophic health care expenses. And more than 90% of health expenditure is incurred in the private sector.

The public sector is only used by patients who do not have medical coverage or people on medical assistance, which leads to the impoverishment of hospitals with a loss of revenue for the latter. Added to this is the fragmentation of health information systems.

The average occupancy rate (AOR) of public hospitals varies from **35–67%**, with an average of 62% [5], which means that almost 4 out of 10 beds are empty. In the private sector, this rate exceeds 85%.

In addition, there is a shortage of human resources, with poor distribution and low retention and motivation of staff in remote areas. The number of doctors is only 7 per 10,000 inhabitants, which is below WHO standards, which recommend 23 doctors per 10,000 inhabitants. It is even lower than in neighboring Maghreb countries, with a ratio of 13 doctors per 10,000 inhabitants in Tunisia and 17 doctors per 10,000 inhabitants in Algeria.

The average productivity of surgeons is 166 operations per year, that is, one operation out of two. As for specialist doctors, they make 789 consultations per year, which corresponds to 3.2 consultations per day. This productivity is never indexed only to the health personnel, the whole system which makes that even if this personnel stays in the hospital for 24 hours, and you lock them up, the working conditions in the public hospital which go from stretcher bearer, the elevator which sometimes breaks down, the unavailability of the operating room. All this means that the number of possible interventions in the public system by the number of public doctors automatically gives us this failure. However, we have today a recognized competence, that our Moroccan doctors are recruited abroad.

The budget of the Ministry of Health and Social Welfare represents only 5.8% of the general state budget, which is still insufficient by international standards. The Abuja Declaration and the World Health Organization (WHO) specify that the state should devote 15 and 12% of its budget to the Ministry of Health, respectively.

Preventive care accounts for only 5% of current health expenditure. Knowing that a health system not based on primary care consumes a lot of budgets, human resources, and infrastructure, for poor results.

The last revision of the national reference rate (NRR) for the reimbursement of drugs and medical procedures dates back to 2006, creating a gap between practitioners' fees and the reimbursement scale that is constantly widening and aggravating the co-payment remaining at the expense of the citizen. Normally, this national reference rate should be revised every three years. In addition, the patient must pay the co-payment, even for those with long-term illnesses. Normally, reimbursement is made differently, depending on whether it is an originator or a generic drug, as follows (agreement between the National Health Insurance Agency, the National Fund for Social Welfare Organizations, and the National Social Security Fund):

- In the absence of a generic drug, the originator is reimbursed according to its purchase price;
- Any generic drug is reimbursed according to its own price;
- In the presence of one or more generics, the reimbursement of the originator is based on the closest generic in terms of purchase price.

Generally, the reimbursement is 80% for the National Fund for Social Welfare and 70% for the National Social Security Fund.

If the beneficiary has applied for a long-term illness (LTI) that has been accepted by a medical examination, he or she will be recognized as having an LTI and will benefit from an advantageous rate, which is 100% for members of the National Fund for Social Welfare Organizations. For members of the National Social Security Fund, this rate is 90% if the service is provided in public hospitals and 85% if it is provided in private hospitals.

For analyses, the reimbursement is 80% for the National Social Security Fund even in the case of LTI and 90% for the National Social Security Fund if the service is provided in the public sector; otherwise, it is 85%.

The drug policy poses a major problem for the health system. The first contact of the Moroccan citizen with the health system is the pharmacy because it is closer and allows him to save a medical consultation. The public selling price (PSP) applied in private pharmacies is set by the Directorate of Medicines and Pharmacy (DMP) according to the benchmark method with seven countries (France, Spain, Belgium, Portugal, Saudi Arabia, Turkey, and the country of origin). This method identifies the cheapest public selling price among the seven countries as mentioned in article 3 of the pricing method of the official bulletin No. 6214–15 Safar 1735 (19-12-2013).

$$\begin{aligned} PSP(\text{Public sale price}) &= \text{Manufacturer's price excluding value added } tax \\ &\quad + \text{Dispensary margin} + \text{Distributor's margin} + \text{Value added } tax \end{aligned}$$

These benchmark countries do not have a similar economic level as Morocco (not the same purchasing power, not the same gross domestic product, etc.)

According to the latest national health accounts of 2018, 45.6% of health expenditure is borne by households, to which must be added 14.1% of medical coverage [1]. In France, they are at 8%, and in Canada and Sweden, they are at 1%. However, despite a drop in direct payments by households compared to previous years, the level recorded is still high compared to internationally recommended standards of less than 25%.

4. Universal coverage: Out of reach or feasible

The question that arises, and which deserves careful consideration, is the following. How will a health system, already marked by numerous failures, be able to absorb 22 million new beneficiaries in order to achieve medical coverage for 100% of the Moroccan population by the end of 2022?

Certainly, with the integration of almost all Moroccans into this system, the system will be faced with an unprecedented increase in demand. This project is worthy and commendable, but it risks being a missed opportunity if we do not change the paradigm, governance, and overall organization of our system upstream to make it more equitable and efficient.

4.1 Accompanying measures

Indeed, Morocco, through the framework law 09–21, has undertaken an overhaul of its health system, based on various accompanying measures:

- First of all, the upgrading of public health care structures, in order to improve the attractiveness of the public hospital so that it can attract not only holders of the medical assistance card but also insured persons.

- The development of public–private partnerships remains unavoidable in order to succeed in this project. The private sector is very active and also heavily involved in the development of infrastructure, in the production of medicines and health technologies, and in their supply. In general, the public sector is overwhelmed by demand, while supply does not follow, hence the importance of mobilizing all resources, whether public or private, in order to rehabilitate hospital supply.

- The strengthening of prevention, early diagnosis, and primary care programs and the revision of the hospital management system with administrative and financial autonomy and an internal and external audit system.

- Efforts to recruit train and improve the working conditions of health staff.

- The introduction of a new governance of the health system with the territorial health grouping. The pilot experiment has already been launched in the Fez-Meknes region in northern Morocco. It is a medical and health care strategy implemented within a territory and serving patient care like the Territorial Hospital Grouping in France. The territorial health grouping is a regional steering instrument that defines the distribution of medical and paramedical resources in the regional territory and the way they are used. It is therefore a tool for reorganizing the supply of care, the aim being to optimize the availability and pooling of human, material, and financial resources between networks and care channels from the ambulatory structures up to the tertiary level; that is, these resources will be put at the service of the population in a territory that creates centers of excellence and not at the level of the structure.

  This territorial grouping requires the creation of an autonomous regional health establishment capitalizing on the university hospital center. The latter will absorb all the regional health establishments to become the leader at the regional level, and its main mission will be to manage all the health establishments and to implement the health policies of the Ministry of Health and Social Protection at the regional level. This means that all 12 regions of Morocco must have a university hospital center; for the moment, the country has only five functional university hospital centers in Casablanca, Rabat, Fez, Marrakech, and Oujda, in addition to three under construction in Tangier, Agadir, and Laâyoune.

- The overhaul of the institutional architecture of the public health system with the transition from a pyramidal system by level to a system of channels and care paths.

- Changing the status of staff and introducing new innovative incentive models such as capped fee-for-service and capitation payments.

  Despite the level of reimbursement, even in the case of long-term conditions, the remaining costs for patients are still high. The revision of the national reference rate is crucial to get closer to the real expenses.

- With a view to harmonizing the effective coverage by the health insurance funds, raising the awareness of the various parties involved (doctors, pharmacists) with regard to the revision of the protocols and therapeutic schemes validated for reimbursement is decisive. In addition, pharmacists should be encouraged to adhere to the third-party payment agreement between the National Health Insurance Agency, the health insurance bodies, and the federation of pharmacists in order to avoid partial reimbursement of medicines after the fact.

- Advocacy for the reduction of drug prices is a big work and awareness that must be done in this sense on the reduction of public selling prices. The Ministry of Health and Social Protection must apply law 17–04, obliging pharmaceutical laboratories domiciled in Morocco to market their medicines after obtaining marketing authorization while respecting the regulatory deadlines. In other words, laboratories that choose to set up in Morocco because of the country's political stability or the cost of labor and to market their medicines abroad must respect the regulations in force after obtaining the marketing authorization given by the Department of Medicines and Pharmacy.

- Introduction of hospital billing within the hospital, similar to what is done in private pharmacies for magistral preparations in order to reduce the hospital bill.

- Funding autonomy based on the health insurance scheme with a total billing model and the introduction of an integrated information system.

4.2 Other challenges

As financing health from traditional tax revenues is not sufficient to meet the needs of the population, effective resource mobilization through increasing the health budget remains necessary. In addition, the rationalization of the use of available resources and the adoption of new financing mechanisms such as the taxation of products harmful to health, increased taxes on airline tickets, foreign exchange transactions, and private services such as telecommunications are already being progressively implemented [6].

Other challenges remain to be met in order to succeed in this project, namely the revision of the national reference tariff, the nomenclature of professional acts and therapeutic protocols, the revision of the pricing policy, the local manufacture of generics, etc.

In addition to the other challenges, the list of reimbursable medicines needs to be further expanded. For medicines that do not yet have a marketing authorization (MA), the pharmaceutical company concerned must obtain an MA, the public selling price

(PPV), and the hospital price (PH), which are set by the Ministry of Health and Social Protection (MHSP) through the Department of Medicines and Pharmacy. Afterward, it applies to the National Health Insurance Agency (NHIA) for reimbursement of the drug.

The list of medicines selected for reimbursement is drawn up by commissions composed of representatives of the MHSP, the health insurance funds, and the NHIA, on the basis of the medical service rendered (SMR) of each medicine. The Transparency Commission (CT) gives the MHSP an opinion on the SMR of a medicine that has already obtained a marketing authorization, with a view to its inclusion or removal from the list of reimbursable medicines.

In order to strengthen the criteria for the reimbursement of medicines, the NHIA has created the Commission for the Economic and Financial Evaluation of Health Products (CEFHP). The latter decides on all applications concerning medicines, by analyzing the economic and financial impact of medicines that have been given a favorable medical service by the CT. This commission decides on all applications concerning medicines, by analyzing the economic and financial impact of medicines that have been given a favorable medical service by the CT.

Can addressing these challenges and the profound overhaul of the national health system make the system more efficient and equitable? In other words, is there a perfect health system?

5. Good health system: Does it exist or not?

The only clear and indisputable evidence is that there is no such thing as a good health system; such a system would be one that manages to connect the four poles of a magic square as shown in **Figure 1**.

First is through the achievement of medical efficiency with better medical outcomes, sound research programs, and good quality of care. The United States is a very good example of medical efficiency, winning more than half of the Nobel Prizes in Medicine,

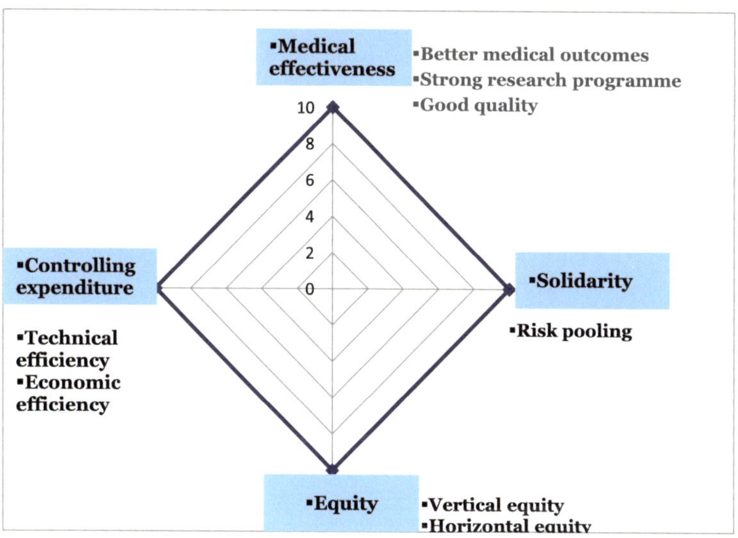

Figure 1.
Source: Chakib Boukhalfa 2022.

making it the most innovative country in the medical field. Add to this the fact that continuing education for doctors in the United States is mandatory in all 50 states and doctors have to revalidate their degrees regularly, but what about solidarity and fairness?

Added to this is the control of expenditure with technical and economic efficiency, linking the labor and capital factor with the contribution to the production of care and the improvement of health status with costs.

Secondly, the preservation of solidarity with a mutualization of risks, that is, the healthy pay for the sick, the active pay for the passive, and the young pay for the elderly.

And finally, there is equity, with the assurance of vertical equity, that is, people should pay different amounts, depending on their ability to pay, and horizontal equity, that is, people should be treated in the same way if they have a similar problem, regardless of their social or geographical origin. France is a good example, but until when.

It is clear that no health system can claim to have the perfect formula, in terms of both equal access to quality care and economic efficiency. Experiences have revealed many flaws within the different health systems, especially in relation to inequalities and inequity [7]. This calls for a project to reform the whole system for better performance.

6. Conclusion

The health problem is a multi-sectoral problem that requires the federation of efforts of all actors and not only the Ministry of Health and Social Welfare. As mentioned in the 1982 Organization for Economic Co-operation and Development report, "Improvement in health status depends on 20% of the health system; the remaining 80% are the external determinants of the system."

To conclude, we could not find a better excerpt from the royal letter addressed to the participants in the celebration of the World Health Day: "Universal health coverage is not an unattainable goal, just as it is not the prerogative of advanced countries alone. Indeed, many experiences have shown, in a tangible way, that this objective is perfectly achievable, whatever the level of development of a country."

As mentioned in the royal letter, the dream of generalizing medical coverage in any country can become a reality. In order to achieve this in its current state, specific efforts must be made, especially in the area of reducing the price of medicines and changing the governance and overall organization of our system. In general, the planning of this project must be carried out on an ongoing basis. Other awareness-raising and accompanying actions must be designed in advance to guarantee the progress made to date and to make the system even more equitable and efficient.

Author details

Chakib Boukhalfa
National School of Public Health, Rabat, Morocco

*Address all correspondence to: chakib.boukhalfa@gmail.com

References

[1] Report 2002. OECD Development Review 2003/1 (n° 4). Investing in Health to Reduce Poverty. Austria: OECD Publishing; 2002. pp. 185-201. ISBN 92-64610091-1

[2] National Health Accounts, Ministry of Health. Morocco: Ministry of Health and Social Protection; 2018

[3] National Health Insurance Agency, Ministry of Health and Social Protection. Morocco: Ministry of Health and Social Protection; 2022

[4] National Population and Family Health Survey (NPFHS), Ministry of Health. Morocco: Ministry of Health and Social Protection; 2018

[5] Health in Figures, Ministry of Health. Morocco: Ministry of Health and Social Protection; 2017

[6] McCoy D, Brikci N. Taskforce on innovative international financing for health systems: What next? Bulletin of the World Health Organization. 2010;**88**(6):478-480. DOI: 10.2471/BLT.09.074419

[7] Polton D. Are our health systems sustainable? Health, Society and Solidarity. 2008;125-135

Chapter 8

Poor Health Care Access in Nigeria: A Function of Fundamental Misconceptions and Misconstruction of the Health System

Vivien O. Abah

Abstract

Health care access in Nigeria is very limited in all dimensions due to factors within and beyond the health system. Misconception of primary health care and poor leadership resulted in a stunted health system development which has failed to align system structures and processes to the goal of achieving universal health access. Improving financial access through compulsory health insurance will not be enough to reverse this status without a holistic primary health care reform to correct the system misconstruction, achieve high-quality health care that is efficient, acceptable to the people and therefore sustainable and capable of driving growth and development for the health system and the country. A primary health care movement consisting of health professionals within the country and the diaspora and other stakeholders is needed to drive this process and overcome the inertia of political leadership in this regard.

Keywords: health care access, primary health care, reform, quality of care, health system organization

1. Introduction

The World Health Organization defines access to health as universal health coverage which means that all people have access to the health services they need, when and where they need them of sufficient quality to be effective, without financial hardship. The goal should include the full range of essential health services, from health promotion to prevention, treatment, rehabilitation and palliative care and beyond to holistic improvement of well-being and quality of life [1]. To achieve universal health care, a nation needs policy-makers committed to investing in universal health coverage, skilled health workers providing high-quality, people-centered care in a health system founded on a strong, people-centered primary health care rooted in the communities they serve [1].

This definition encompasses 2 major pillars of health care access: financial access and the quality of the services accessed. The emphasis on quality of care is

IntechOpen

very important because it determines the capacity of the service to deliver "health" to the users.

The reformed primary health care is defined as first-contact, comprehensive, continuing, coordinated, person centered care delivered to the individual within the context of his family and community through a defined regular provider. It is care delivered by professional health care providers in teams that take primary responsibility for the health of defined population of people and their community. It therefore has the competence to offer effective, appropriate and safe care to all patients for most of the problems they have most of the time at first contact thereby achieving comprehensive care which integrates personal curative, preventive, promotive and palliative with family and community engagement. Responsibility for a defined population of people makes them the regular source of care and entry point into the health system therefore offering continuous care over the life course with increased mutual knowledge and understanding between the patient and providers strengthening provider- patient relationship which facilitates trust, empathy, person-centeredness and therefore efficacy of care. The primary care provider takes responsibility for coordinating the health care needs of the patients when specialist care beyond the first contact is required and maintains on going care after the referral has been accessed. This serves to entrench quality care, efficiency, increased safety, individual utilization and community ownership and participation. It serves as the foundation of the health system. This mode of primary care has been evidenced provide high-quality care to the population, achieving the desired health outcomes. The undergirding principle of the reformed PHC is that it serves as a means of providing the highest attainable level of health for all citizens maximizing equity and solidarity, integrating citizens' expectations with structures and processes to attain them, i.e., guided by responsiveness [2].

Globally, about 50% of people do not have access to health care and about 100 M people are pushed into poverty every year due to catastrophic health expenditures [1].

All over the world, access to health care and quality of care have been on the increase in a sustained pattern as evidenced by the Global Healthcare Access and Quality Index Scores: from 37.6/100 in 1900 to 42.4 in 2000 and 54.4 in 2016. However, around 7.3 billion people are unable to access all the essential health services that they need, and it is estimated that in 137 countries around 8.6 million excess deaths occurred in 2016 as a consequence of poor access to quality health care, particularly in low- and middle-income countries as at 2017 [3].

The concept of access to health care has been variously defined and conceptualized in dimensions by different authors to enable its study, understanding and measurement. The Penchansky definition of access in 5 As is very commonly used and will be combined with the Levesque's framework for this discussion.

Levesque's framework defines access as the opportunity or ability to identify or perceive a health need, seek, reach, pay/obtain, or use health care and to ensure the fulfilment of the needs for these services. This framework is chosen because of its' comprehensive approach incorporating factors attributable to the health delivery system, the social determinants of health and the patient. The framework sets out the process of health seeking to include a continuum from the existence of a health need to perception of the need and desire to seek care, the care seeking action, ability to reach the source of care, utilizing care and deriving the desired outcomes.

Ability to perceive a health need is determined by personal factors as health literacy, beliefs, trust and expectations of health facilities. Health system (HS) factors as the delivery of transparency, outreach, information and screening to the populace impacts this capacity. This is equated to the Penchansky dimension of Approachability.

Seeking health care is determined by social determinants of health (SDH) factors as personal and social values, culture, gender and autonomy of the patient. HS factors impacting this include professional values of health care providers norms culture and gender which impact the patient's perception of the available health facility and services. This depicts the Penchansky dimension of Acceptability.

Health seeking action is determined by SDH factors as living environments, transport, mobility and social support and by HS factors as geographic location of services, opening hours, accommodation, appointment systems. This corresponds to the Penchansky dimension of Availability and Accommodation.

Health care utilization or ability to pay is determined by SDH factors as income, assets, social capital and health insurance and by HS factors as direct, indirect and opportunity costs of service utilization and is equivalent to the Penchansky dimension of Affordability.

Deriving appropriate/desired outcomes from health services which includes satisfaction, health and economic derivatives for individuals and populations is determined by SDH factors as empowerment, information, adherence, care giver support and by HS factors as technical and interpersonal quality of services, adequacy, coordination and continuity of care. All these are equated to the Penchansky dimension of Appropriateness.

It is necessary for this discussion to use this comprehensive systemic framework that incorporates the interconnections between SDH factors with HS factors given the fact that due to poor development in all sectors, these factors are generally negative thereby constituting barriers to access to health [4].

2. The Nigeria Health System

- Nigeria population: 217,373,637M [5].
- 36 states and the federal capital territory.
- 774 local government areas.
- 52.0% lives in urban areas [6].
- Health Budget % total budget: 5.97% (2022) NGN3,453/capita [7].
- Health Expenditure % GDP: 3.03% less than Ethiopia and Ghana [8]
- Government Expenditure /capita: Nigeria; 15.95 USD, Ghana: 40.24 USD Ethiopia: 22.70USD, Canada: 70.17USD
- Private expenditure per capita: Nigeria: 71.30%, Ghana:48.48%, Ethiopia:43.19%, Chile 49.08%, Canada:29.83%.

3. Health indices

- Life expectancy in Nigeria: 2021
- Total: 60.87, Males: 59.07, Female: 62.78

- Neonatal mortality (approximately in 2016/2017) 40/1000. Infant mortality: 80/1,000 Underfive mortality: 120/1000 (NSHDP II)
- Maternal mortality rate:800/100,000 (approximate 2015, NSHDP II)

4. Distribution of Health Facilities as at 2015 (NSHDP II)

Type of health facility Public Private Total

- Primary Health Centers: 30,098 (Public: 21,808, Private: 8,290)
- Secondary Health Facilities: 3,992 (Public: 969 Private: 3,023)
- Tertiary Health Facilities: 86 (Public:86, Private: 10)
- **Total 34,176**

5. Distribution of health manpower

- Doctors in Nigeria 2022 [9]
- Doctors 24,600. Population ratio, 1:8,836.
- Dentists: 1,400. population ratio, 1: 155,267. Required at ratio of 1 doctor /600 population: 362,289 doctors. Deficit: 338,289
- Nurses: 249,566 Population ratio 1:1,677 (NHSDP II,2015)
- Senior CHEWs: Total: 42,938 population ratio 1:28,256 (NHSDP II,2015)
- Junior CHEWs: Total: 28,548 population ratio 1: 5,914 (NHSDP II,2015)

The Nigerian health system is organized in three tiers: primary, secondary and tertiary care levels. The primary health centers are deployed at the grass roots in the ward health system which locates a primary health center at each political ward (9,560 wards) to be run by the local government authority. Secondary health care is delivered at the general hospitals run by the state governments and each is deployed to cover several local governments. The tertiary hospitals are run by the federal government and offer tertiary care and health manpower training in teaching hospitals and federal medical centers [6]. NSHDP II.

The primary health care delivery system consists of pyramids of health facilities in the villages/neighborhoods (health posts covering 500 persons), primary health clinics(one per group of villages covering 2000–5000 persons) and the primary health centers at the apex covering each political ward consisting of 10–20,000 persons. The health providers at these facilities are deployed such that health posts are manned by community health extension workers, clinics are manned by a nurse/midwife and the health centers by a doctor or nurse where available. Linkages to the secondary and tertiary health facilities are affected via a two-way referral system.

The system was planned to be the basis of the health system of the country and a foundation for further growth and development of the system. This system was to deliver the ward minimum package of health services (WMPHS) representing the purposed essential package of health services (EPHS) for Nigerians. Health care utilization is designed to begin at the primary health center as entry point and for cases beyond the capacity of the personnel and facilities to be referred upward to the secondary and then to the tertiary care levels as warranted [10].

Generally, majority of the PHC facilities are in deplorable condition. The evidence of the poor structural and process quality of services is widely documented [6]. A review of PHC facilities in 5 states and the federal capital territory provides evidence on the state of the facilities as shown below [11].

Geographical distribution: Only 22% met stipulated catchment population coverage range of one facility to 1–36 communities (1 facility to 20,000 people)) and at a distance from community of 1–49 km.

State of the buildings: 38.4% facilities required major renovations while 34% required minor renovations.

Forty Nine percent had cracked walls, 50.7% had cemented floors, 21.9% had rough floors and a large proportion (58.9%) had leaking roofs.

Security: only 24.7% of the facilities had perimeter fencing.

Power supply: 38.4% were connected to the national electricity grid, Solar power: 8.2%. generator: 23.3% with only few having functional generators or fuel to run them.

Water Supply: only 30% used motorized bore hole, 7 facilities depended on rain, 8 facilities on surface waters like streams, rivers and dams, 16 used wells. Of these only 65% of facilities have a water outlet within 500 m. 5 facilities had zero source of water.

Toilet facilities: 31%: had no toilet facility. 25% used pit latrines, 16% used piped sewer system. Only 23% had a flush system.

Emergency ambulance vehicle: only 5.5% had emergency ambulance, 2.7% had emergency transportation system including motorcycles and car.

Referral system: 11% had referral system.

Majority (79.1%) had access roads, only 24.7% were tarred and in variable conditions.

Accommodation for staff, only 30.1% had some form of accommodation for some staff. All were in deplorable conditions and none met the stipulated regulatory (NPHCDA) standards.

Communication: Only 31.5% facilities had a functional means of communication.

Information technology facilities: only 2.7% facilities had functional computers / internet.

Basic medical equipment like stethoscopes, sphygmomanometers, thermometers, weighing scales and infusion sets were available in at least 50% of facilities but others required for simple emergency care like oxygen cylinders, nebulizers, ambubags, basic suturing, etc., were not available in majority of facilities.

Non-professional health manpower (CHEWs) was in very short supply obviously limiting service availability and operating hours.

The pattern of utilization and service availability was in favor of immunizations, antenatal care and deliveries in keeping with programmatic interventions for the target populations.

Given the state of these facilities, their capacity to deliver "health care" is obviously questionable. The PHCs are often the only health facilities available in rural areas and 48% of Nigeria is rural, this therefore depicts the health care access to this population.

6. Misconception of Primary Health Care in Nigeria

The ward health system was developed in response to the Alma-ata primary health care (PHC) reform in 1978 and was instituted as the basis of the health system in the first comprehensive national health development policy 1988 and remains the structure for health care delivery till date [10]. The WHO declaration of primary health care as a means of achieving health for all in 1978 was undergirded by the rationale that at that time, the global disease burden was dominated by preventable communicable disease for which low cost interventions had a high impact relative to cost of investment, many countries were yet to define a viable and stable structure for health delivery and investments were skewed towards curative rather than preventive medicine, the importance of social determinants of disease and multisectoral collaboration for health was underemphasized [2].

The Alma Ata declaration therefore aimed to put forward a set of values and principles to guide the development of health systems by placing national and global solidarity for health on the front burner and persuading countries especially in LMIC to take ownership of responsibility for the health of their populations and invest in health. Hence the main thrust of the PHC was development of PHC as the basis of the health delivery vehicle for health systems such as to provide access to services at grassroots with community participation and ownership, and services targeted at community and personal preventive care, maternal and child health care, treatment of common diseases and injuries and provision of essential drugs. Globally, countries responded and reformed their health systems in the spirit of primary care. Developed countries reformed and improved on their delivery of holistic care integrating preventive, curative and rehabilitative care attaining high population coverage and improved health indices. Low- and middle-income countries (LMICs) evolved differently with very poor outcome. In Nigeria as in most LMIC, PHC was fundamentally misconceived as an intervention program to deliver basic health services for priority diseases to the rural poor with the main thrust as community preventive health care and that personal curative care needed was of a basic nature not requiring professional health care providers and technology. The focus was therefore on priority segments of the population: women and children and those suffering from conditions like tuberculosis, guinea worm, etc., for which donor programs were available. This approach defined the governments' perspective to health system development: intervention to the rural poor using non-professional health workers for priority diseases defined by the global donors thereby denying majority of the population access to health care. This misconceived approach to health care and health system development failed to deliver health to the populations and coupled with poor leadership and massive corruption led to massive waste of resources, stunted health system development and abysmal health indices for the nation.

7. Failure of the PHC

The guiding policy for health delivery in Nigeria, the National Strategic Health Development Plan II (NSHDP II) states that the goal of the policy is "to strengthen Nigeria's health system, particularly the Primary Health Care sub system, to deliver quality, effective, efficient, equitable, accessible, affordable, acceptable and comprehensive health care services to all Nigerians". The PHC system was deployed to the grass roots but geographical access did not translate to access to health care as majority (80%) of these facilities were not utilized by the populations [6]. The myriad of reasons for this included, perceived poor quality of services, principally due to the fact that available health care providers were not capable of delivering competent care to meet the needs of the populations. The expressed health needs of people that make them seek care (which are mostly curative and beyond the prescribed preventive care) require the expertise of professional care providers: doctors, nurses, pharmacists, etc., and not the community health extension workers (CHEWs) found in most PHC. Poor utilization consequently resulted in economic unviability of these facilities and abandonment by both the populations and the government and their dilapidation.

This was noted by the WHO PHC review and reform document to be the case in countries utilizing low cadre health care providers. It is unlike in high-income countries where primary care was provided by specialist physicians with competence to offer high-quality comprehensive first-contact care thereby facilitating early detection of diseases and appropriate management, preventing complications and mortality. There is therefore a fundamental mismatch between the needs and aspirations of the people and the services that were provided for them: failure of people centered care. This has been attributed by the WHO as the principal cause of the failure of the progress of health systems in LMICs. It is the fundamental cause of the failure of PHC in Nigeria. Even the poor recognize their need for professional quality health care and are no longer content to be recipients of intervention programs that cater to selected diseases. The NSHDP II acknowledges this and states that despite previous reform efforts and *investments, ..."efforts at health system strengthening have not had the desired effect*, resulting in limited health care coverage and persistently poor health status of the population". The 2018 strategic health plan goal of provision of high-quality health care for all Nigerians via the PHC is in itself a contradiction reflecting the lack of understanding of the misalignment of the current concept, structure and reality of the outcome of the PHC system in the country to this goal. There have been two national strategic health development plans since 2008, the 2010–2015 and 2018–2022 in which the system has been reviewed, the failures documented but reform has been only on paper and without addressing the crucial causes of failure. The WHO 2008 report on PHC reform was referenced in these plans but none of its recommendations were included in the plans [2]. Poor leadership and entrenched lack of responsiveness and responsibility have resulted in refusal to reform the system based on local evidence and the WHO reform agenda.

8. Poor leadership

The principle of social justice which makes the right to health a fundamental human right to be guaranteed by government has been neglected in Nigeria due to poor leadership in government and also within the health sector. The Nigerian government did not institutionalize the right to health of citizens until the enactment of the National Health Act of 2014 [12]. The laissez -faire attitude to health care is evident in poor funding, policy enactment and implementation resulting in the persistent approach to health as a commodity for which the populations have individual personal responsibility. The PHCs are statutorily under the governance of the local government authority which is non-functional as a tier of government in Nigeria. The NPHCDA at national level has been supervising and funding the PHC through very opaque mechanisms directly and via the state PHCDAs. Poor leadership has left this system uncorrected despite the impact of this misconstruction on the performance and accountability of PHC system.

9. Corruption and mismanagement

There is an endemic pervasive culture of corruption in Nigeria which is largely responsible for the state of the health system and nation. The misconception and failure to reform the PHC in line with the WHO recommendations is based on this. Corruption has made it impossible for the leadership both within the health system and government to walk the talk and altruistically work to build a system that can provide access to health care for the population. The lack of sense of social justice undergirds the misconception that PHC is a program for the poor, and the refusal to reform the system despite the overwhelming evidence of its failure and rejection and the knowledge of the availability of the WHO strategy for reform. Their knowledge and rejection of the poor quality of care in Nigeria is evidenced by the whopping 1.6B USD capital flight from Nigeria spent on medical tourism annually especially by the political class [13]. Monumental graft in the system has consumed the available funding and greatly accelerated the collapse of the system.

Poor funding: The health budget has been consistently below 5% of national budget contrary to the fact of Nigeria being a signatory to charters recommending more than this (Abuja declaration recommending 15%). This performance is less than most countries of comparable income. The 2022 health budget was 4.3% of total budget amounting to about N3,453 per capita [7]. An amount that is incapable of providing access to health care for anyone. The dependence on donor funding for the priority diseases and programs may be a factor since these conditions are also the ones tracked for health system performance.

Policy development: Government ownership of the responsibility for health of her citizens warrants that health status, risk factors, morbidity and mortality trends are tracked to develop priorities and guide policy development but in Nigeria it is not so. Health priorities are determined by global agencies and donors and implementation is entirely to satisfy the conditions set for the vertical programs. This has often resulted in very poor performance of these programs, inefficient use of resources and poor sustainability. Also, it has contributed to the stunted development of the health system as the focus is on vertical programs targeted at segments of the population to satisfy global concerns but not on holistic health delivery for the entire population. The failure of the numerous vertical programs and their fragmenting impact on the system led to the development of the Primary Health Care Under One Roof initiative [14]. This aimed to integrate the multiple programs under one management, eliminate duplicate funding, staffing, facilities and competition but has not succeeded in achieving better results for the programs or improved performance for the system. Vertical stand-alone programs are expensive and inefficient and need to be mainstreamed into a well- structured PHC system that is capable of offering comprehensive first-contact care to all segments of the population [2]. This is also noted by the WHO as a major contributor to the failure of health systems in LMICs [2].

Data management culture and research: poor sense of responsibility for the system and commitment to its development is also evidenced in poor data management culture which has permeated the entire system evidenced by lack of current Nigerian Government date for all indicators within and beyond the health system. Lack of value for the use of data to guide policy and decisions has resulted in a culture of disregard for accuracy, timeliness and sanctity of data collection and management. It is generally regarded as only necessary to be seen to meet program tasks. There is a wealth of research evidence as to the poor performance and community rejection of PHC but this fact has not deterred the government from persisting in its' pursuit as the basis of health care delivery system in Nigeria. The National Strategic Health Development Plans acknowledge these evidences, the failure of government to implement measures to address the problems and yet insists on "strengthening" the existing PHC system to deliver quality health care to all citizens.

The health indices of Nigeria have remained persistently deplorable, worse than peer countries, among the worst globally and in contradiction to her great potentials. This is well documented in the national strategic health plans (NSHDP II) including the fact that there is no tangible effort to redeem the situation and adopt the WHO reform strategy. This approach to PHC has stunted the development of the health system and thus denied Nigerians access to health care.

10. Misconstruction and misalignments

A health system is defined as all the resources, actors and institutions related to the financing, regulation and provision of activities whose primary intent is to improve or maintain health [15]. The intrinsic goals of a health system are to provide good health, responsiveness and financial fairness for the population. The health of the population as a primary outcome of the system should reflect the health of individuals throughout life including both premature mortality, non-fatal health outcomes and the distribution of these in the population and reduction of inequalities. The health system structure and processes must therefore be aligned to achieve these goals. The key functional components of the system must therefore include institutions to provide for financing, service delivery, resource generation and stewardship with these institutions working in synergy to achieve the goals of the system for society. Policy, strategic design and implementation must therefore be aligned to the achievement of these goals facilitated by a framework for evaluation and reform over time.

The construction of the health system in Nigeria and its capacity to provide health and access to same is discussed in this context.

11. Financial access

National Health budgeting:

- The financing function of the HS in Nigeria is one obvious cause of poor access to care.

- The national budget allocation for health at average of 5% is consistently below the WHO recommendation of 15% and less than many Sub Saharan African countries despite having greater economic means [6].

The National Health Act (2014) established the responsibility of government for the health of Nigerians and instituted the basic health care provision fund (BHCPF) to provide the essential package of health services (EPHS) or basic health care package (BHCP) for the citizens [12]. The BHCPF is derived from 1% of consolidated revenue of the federal government and the EPHS stipulates the minimum package of health services that every citizen is entitled to. The principle of establishing EPHS in a health system is to serve as a tool for guaranteeing equitable access to health. It should be designed with specific funding and delivery mechanism for quality health care, plans for upgrading of the package and also serves as a means to guide budgeting for health. The EPHS as designed in Nigeria contains the provision of water and sanitation and six personal health interventions: four maternal and child interventions and one urinalysis and one blood pressure measurement for others not in the maternal and child bracket [16]. The content of this package represents the basic obligation of the government to citizens for health and demonstrates the minimal consideration to achieve health for majority of citizens. In Nigeria water is provided by individual private bore holes and government action in this regard is minimal. Sanitation in urban areas is contracted by government and paid for by citizens. At a birth rate of 37/1000, the estimated number of pregnant women and infants in a given year is 7.6 million mothers and 7.6 million babies approximately, covering only 7% of the population is covered. Also, maternal and child health services are already covered by primary health care services funded by NPHCDA budgets and donors in multiple vertical programs. The provision of the funding of reproductive, maternal, neonatal, child and adolescent health (RMNCAH) services in the BHCPF amounts to a duplication and therefore renders the stewardship of the funds opaque.

The provision of one blood pressure check and one urinalysis for those outside the maternal and child target population cannot be equated to a health care package thereby confirming that the government does not feel obligated to give her citizens access to health care. It is in fact a travesty of responsibility. The content of the EPHS contradicts the principles under girding the design of EPHS as it neither provides health care nor equity for the population [2, 17]. This is unlike developed countries where the EHP content is comprehensive and other countries in LMIC category like Ethiopia which includes curative care for non-communicable diseases (NCDs) in the EPHS and recognizes that water and sanitation are delivered by other sectors outside the health services [18].

The stewardship of the BHCPF further jeopardizes its' capacity to meet its' goals. The fund is designed to be deployed through 3 routes: the National Health Insurance Scheme: (50%) for delivery of EPHS to the poor, NPHCDA: (45% for primary health care) for the provision of vaccines, essential drugs and consumables, maintenance of equipment and facilities and development of human resources for health. Federal ministry of health (FMoH) is allocated 5% of the funds for interventions to reduce mortality from road traffic accidents on 5 most dangerous routes in the country [16]. This is a clear departure from the stated intention of the BHCPF in the national health act. The operationalization document of the BHCPF clearly acknowledged that the entire fund cannot provide the health expenditure per capita and cannot buy any real basic package of health care and should therefore be targeted at providing the EPHS for the poor and yet the fund is split to include the FMOH for provision of emergency services through an unfeasible and opaque mechanism. Also, the funds given to the NPHCDA to cover services already previously provided for creates a duplication which is unaccounted for unlike in Uganda where such overlaps resulted in closure of vertical stand-alone programs for TB and leprosy and their incorporation into mainstream services [18].

Health insurance coverage. The capacity to purchase health is a major barrier to access where financial risk protection is lacking. Out of pocket expenditure for health at 71% is one of the highest among peer countries [8]. With nearly half of the citizens living below the poverty line, significant proportions of the population delay seeking health care, utilize quacks, or forfeit care altogether [19]. Effort at establishing universal health coverage via the national health insurance scheme (NHIS) has been in operation since 2005 but has so far covered only 13.5 million people (7%) [20]. The NHIS is a social health insurance scheme and has five major schemes targeting the formal sector employees (FSSHIP), students in tertiary institutions (TSSHIP) vulnerable groups (VGSHIP), informal sector via voluntary schemes, (VCSHIP) community-based insurance (CBI). The federal government funds FSSHIP and TSSHIP which have gained reasonable coverage among the populations targeted (government employees and corporate organizations staff) for these 2 schemes accounting for the 13.5 M people so far covered. The informal sector and community-based schemes which cover most of the population do not receive any government funds and do not have any specific mechanisms to ensure enrolment. The vulnerable group scheme provides for the same health benefit plan as the FSSHIP to be funded by government but has not gained much traction due to the lack of a clear funding mechanism, no reliable data base and mechanism to ensure their enrolment. However, in July, this year (2022) the Federal Government of Nigeria (FGN) announced the signing into law of a new act making health insurance compulsory for all citizens and residents of Nigeria, the National Health Insurance Act 2022 (amendment) also established the National Health Insurance Scheme as the National Health Insurance Authority. A specific funding mechanism for the VGSHIP was also announced to be derived from telecom tax, the basic health care provision fund (BHCPF) and donations. It is expected to cover 83 million Nigerians (43% of the population) and therefore increase the breadth of health insurance coverage of the population [21, 22]. However, a major challenge to achieving this coverage is the stewardship of these funds and accountability of the process of enrolment.

This concern is demonstrated by the fact that the fund was released for the first time in 2019 to the tune of 56 BN and is said to have been deployed to 7,250 health centers for rehabilitation and to cover the NHIS enrolment of about 1,042,890 indigent people of which 753,999 have started receiving the EPHS [23]. This reflects the contradiction in the operationalization of the BHCPF aiming to provide EPHS to the poor via the NHIS, at variance with the NHIS provision that vulnerable group (VGSHIP) enrollees will receive same health benefit plans (HBP) entitled in the FSSSHIP. The achievement of financial access to health care for the vulnerable group via this funding is dependent on if their enrolment entitles them to the same health benefit plan as the FSSHIP or limited to the content of EPHS. This clarification is necessary as there is inconsistency in the announcements of the minister for health and the director general of the NHIA regarding this [20, 23].

Operationalizing the VGSHIP necessitates the consolidation of the entire funds into the NHIA to provide HBP cover for the vulnerable group and therefore avoid duplication and improve the efficiency of resource utilization in the spirit of stewardship.

The community-based health insurance scheme is targeted at rural dwellers who are also mostly poor. They are required to form contributory groups, engage a health management organization to manage the funds and negotiate their HBP with a health management organization (HMO). This scheme receives no funding from government. Many challenges have impeded the deepening of the coverage of this target population: poverty of the target population, poor knowledge of the existence of the scheme, poor community organization and participation and poor quality of available health services in rural health facilities (primary health centers). The poor funding of this scheme from the contributors makes the scheme unviable business for the HMOs, limits the value of the coverage they can receive and therefore limits access to care. However, the VGSHIP will absorb a significant proportion of this population. The government needs to provide a scheme to subsidize the enrolment of those not covered by the VGSHIP in keeping with government's obligation to meet their right to health especially now that health insurance has been made compulsory and as done in other countries [24].

The coverage for the informal sector workers (Voluntary Contributors Health Insurance Scheme VCSHIP) which includes a significant proportion of the population who are engaged in small and medium scale enterprises has also not gained much breath attributed to poor awareness and knowledge of the scheme.

12. Health delivery system

The reformed PHC system empanels individuals, their families and communities with specific primary health care teams led by specialist physicians [2, 25]. This delivery structure enables the system to be accountable for the health of every citizen, allows for regulation of quality of care and facilitates cost effectiveness and efficiency of the system thereby achieving universal access. The health system of the UK, France, Canada, Australia, the Netherlands and Germany are structured as such and their health indices are evidence of its' success. The basis of the health system in these countries is the primary care provider team led by the family physician, general practitioner, primary care internist, or primary care pediatrician [2, 26]. They take care of most of the health needs of most of the population most of the time serving as the gateway to secondary and tertiary care in a coordinated approach [26]. Majority of the doctors in these countries are specialists with a high density of other professional health workers working in integrated teams within systems that span from the community to the hospitals [26]. Quality of care is a priority established on evidence-based practices [26]. Commitment to high-quality care and population outcomes drives the system to set high standards of care using the most efficient solutions in a responsive and responsible manner ensuring equity and solidarity in the spirit of primary health care. Health manpower planning is prioritized and is coordinated from training to employment, distribution and retention. Health budgets are significant proportions of the total GDP, access in ensured via health insurance and out of pocket expenditures are minimal.

The primary health care performance initiative (PHCPI) framework integrates the components of the health system into a framework showing the directionality and interplay of components leading to the achievement of the goals of the system. It demonstrates that achieving the goal of the system is critically determined by the structures, organization and processes linking them.

Some critical components of the framework are totally lacking in our system contributing to the misconstruction and poor foundation for development. These components include quality management infrastructure and social accountability mechanisms, population health management (local priority setting and empanelment) high-quality primary care (first-contact accessibility, continuity, comprehensiveness, coordination and person-centered care), team-based care organization, performance measurement and management. Some components of the outcomes domain are also lacking (responsiveness, equity, efficiency and resilience of health system) all leading to poor health status of the population. This framework emphasizes on the critical importance of the service delivery component which determines the interaction between people and the system thereby leading to outputs.

The misconception of PHC and misconstruction resulting in inability to functionally link system, inputs and service delivery domains of the PHC system to the goal of achieving health for the population made the health delivery system ineffective and inefficient ab initio. The structures including health posts, clinics and primary health centers had at its core goal the programmatic intervention for a small but vulnerable segment of the population in response to donor determined priorities and not quality health care for the entire population.

13. Human resources for health

The most fundamental reason for the failure of the PHC was the lack of professional health care providers, especially doctors to render the services needed by the people. In recognition of this the NSHDPII made human resources for health a major objective of the strategic plan with the goal to *"have in place the right number, skill mix of competent, motivated, productive and equitably distributed health work force for optimal and quality health care services provision"*. The NSHDP II also acknowledges that health manpower development: training, deployment and retention have not received any strategic efforts from government.

Health manpower planning: There is no tangible effort at evaluating the health human resources needed and aligning this with training priorities, employment and retention. There is no reliable data on the number of physicians, nurses or other health workers in the country. All available estimates show that there are insufficient numbers of all cadres of workers with provider population ratios far below the WHO recommendations as discussed above and there is no government action in this regard despite clear documentation as a major objective for health sector development.

Training: health manpower training across all cadres is hindered by the general decay in the educational sector. Unfortunately, the educational system is suffering a similar neglect with incessant industrial actions, dilapidated facilities, low-quality educational processes and inconsistent graduate turn outs due to major interruptions of the academic calendars. It is estimated that at the rate of 3,500 doctors produced per year, it will take Nigeria over a hundred years to produce the 363,000 doctors required to meet the WHO physician-population ratio of 1:600 at our current population of about 218M. There is a staggering deficit of about 338,000 physicians in Nigeria. Primary health care in developed countries is delivered by specialist physician led teams and majority of doctors in these climes are specialized. In Nigeria majority of doctors are not specialized. There is no correlation between health manpower training output and the needs of the health sector. The only effort at manpower development to fill service needs has been at the level of CHEWs via the task shifting and task sharing policy. The CHEWs are being trained to upgrade their capacity to deliver curative services in the primary health centers using standing order protocols in effort to sustain the failed system. Evidence from the review of the PHC has shown that in a survey of 73 PH centers, not one of them had the standing order and that the accuracy of identification of clinical diagnostic entities was about 37% [11, 27]. Among the CHEWs, major challenges noted to impede their work and cause low morale was the lack of professional clinical support and leadership [27]. The persistence of childhood and maternal mortality indices at deplorable levels does not beg further explanation. The gross deficit of professional health manpower results in low technical quality of care ab initio denying majority of Nigerians access to health care.

Deployment: deployment of health manpower should be based on population density with the aim of having adequate numbers and variety of professionals to provide required services. There is no effort in this direction in Nigeria contrary to the strategic plans which made it a major objective to provide the right mix and numbers of health manpower to provide quality health services to all Nigerians. Also, a dysfunctional work culture in the country has resulted in absenteeism in the workplace further worsening the manpower availability situation. Health workers across all cadres are well known to be functionally absent from their jobs limiting hours of service, increasing waiting times in health facilities and creating major barriers to access to health services. Rejection of rural postings due to poor conditions of living is another problem and even when these postings are accepted, the workers arrange to live in the urban centers and be available at limited times in the rural facilities resulting in functional shut down of the facilities they serve and limitation of access to care.

Retention: The laissez faire attitude of the government in this regard has been monumentally detrimental to the development of the health system. The misconception of primary care as basic interventions for the poor to be delivered by non-professional work force probably undergirds this attitude. There are frequent protracted industrial actions within the health sector over work conditions with the hospitals crippled, citizens denied access to care with consequent morbidity and mortality [28]. The government assumes very contentious positions in these disputes and their functionaries have often posited that Nigeria has enough doctors even in the face of critical painful evidence to the contrary calling to question their sense of responsibility on their jobs and to the nation. The consequent mass flight of health manpower to the developed countries has worsened in recent times with about 9,000 doctors leaving in the last 2 years and many more seeking to leave [29]. It is estimated that of the over 75,000 registered doctors in Nigeria only about 24,000 are still in the country including retired doctors [9].

14. Quality of care

The WHO has made it clear that low-quality care is expensive and dangerous [30]. The national strategic health plans and all other health policy documents profusely make quality health care a central goal to be pursued. This is not aligned to any structures and processes that can evaluate and implement quality of care in the system.

Hitherto in our country, failure of PHC has always been premised on poor funding by the government but another argument presents itself in the widespread rejection of these facilities. This rejection has been premised on the perceived poor-quality contingent on the non- professional providers available and their lack of capacity to deal with the health needs of the people and their communities. The facilities failed to offer people centered care.

The mix of non-professional service providers and dilapidated facilities in the health centers are fundamental recipes for poor-quality care and expectedly poor outcomes as evident in Nigeria. A fundamental misconstruction of the system is the lack of a quality management framework resulting in lack of a quality management mind-set and culture among the health care providers and other workers across all strata within and beyond the health system. This is unlike in developed countries where the institutions for managing quality of care are in built critical components of the system empowered to set and enforce standards, e.g., the Care Quality Commission, and NHS Improvement in the UK [26]. These bodies engage professionals, conduct research and develop evidence which are used to guide clinical care and health care priorities. This is critically absent in our system. There is no synergy between the health professionals and the government in this regard. Standards of care are not set within our local realities and resources and the ones copied from developed countries are not monitored or enforced. There is no data on safety of care and it is well known that majority of Nigerians receive inappropriate or even dangerous or unsafe care in hospitals. There are no reliable data on these problems and there is no action in the government or professional organizations to address this. Standards are set only in the regulation documents for registration or periodic reaccreditation for which the facilities are well "informed and prepared." The quality of provider patient interactions and clinical care delivery is completely at the discretion of the provider and only the clients who are empowered seek redress in formal complaints and litigations in a slow and cumbersome judicial system. Quality of care management is critical for the efficiency of the system in attaining its goals. Quality of care frameworks facilitate the development and scaling of best practices ensuring that benefit is equitably distributed, harm is minimized and cost is contained.

Technical and process quality standards setting and regulation are necessarily a function of professional governance enshrined in the professional codes. In Nigeria, the health professions have not been active in engaging, setting and monitoring of the quality of care and practice. Currently there is an unfortunate mistrust of the professions by the populace resulting from multiple factors including the existing exploitative private practices, frequent strike actions with hospital shut downs, poor provider patient interactions and numerous anecdotal reports of questionable care. This has been attributed to the widespread disillusionment and breakdown of ethics in society. However, of note is the significant lack of quality of care and system-based practice as important entities in the curricula of training of health professionals, compounded by lack of quality management framework in the health system. This has resulted in the production of health manpower that is not oriented to the goals of the system, their responsibility and critical leadership roles in its' development, sustenance and outcomes. It is reflected in the endemic subsidiarity in the attitude of individuals, each specialty and professional group with deeply entrenched rivalries that hinder team work and jeopardize quality of care [31]. It has had very adverse impact on the development of the professions limiting their capacity to study disease conditions and develop modalities of care that are suited to our local experience, problems and resources. This is a crucial fundamental building block for effective and efficient care systems as exists in developed countries. The professionals are left with the sense that copying the protocols of care from developed countries is impossible given our limitations but yet unable to develop sustainable alternatives further increasing job frustration and professional unfulfillment. These factors contribute to emigration of health workers. They also result in large performance gaps in the quality of care delivered, development of expertise in care and failure to lay foundations for the system to develop. The performance gaps exist because, due to lack of commitment to a quality management culture, the available limited resources are not put to the best possible use thereby delivering outcomes that are worse than need be. This is a function of professional governance but given the endemic lack of leadership culture in the country, resistance to innovation and poor work culture, the development of professionalism has been stunted.

User perception of quality has also resulted in inefficient use of the system resources. Rejection of PHC services and lack of coordination of care results in self-referral to tertiary institutions in search of quality and ethical care. Most tertiary hospitals are inundated with primary and secondary care conditions leading to overcrowding, long waiting times and underutilization and development of specialist resources [32].

15. Timeliness

User perception of poor quality of care is an important determinant of choice of provider and facility. Waiting time is a major barrier to access to health. Studies have shown that waiting time in Nigerian hospitals can be as long as 6–9 hours [33, 34]. Long waiting times are the result of poor management of patient arrival patterns and coordination of service points. Most public hospitals receive large patient turnouts which overwhelm the available staff and result in long waiting times. Patients decry this scenario and it is one of the major reasons for non- utilization of teaching hospitals hindering access to care. This is despite acknowledging that reliable higher technical quality care is available in teaching hospitals. Unfortunately, due to very poor commitment to responsiveness there is no systemic effort to address this. Simple appointment systems to manage patient arrivals have not been instituted. There is scarcely any public hospital with a telephone number on which they can be reached for anything including emergencies. The COVID-19 experience has failed to change this despite the Nigerian Center for Disease Control (NCDC) protocols requiring that patients with symptoms should call their health care providers before going to the hospital. Long waiting time also contributes to delayed presentation to hospital increasing morbidity and mortality.

Access has so far been discussed with reference to primary care as it is the basis of the health system. The situation with secondary and tertiary care is not more favorable and is largely impeded by similar factors. Availability of highly technical care for such conditions as cancer, stroke, myocardial infarction, etc., is very poor in public tertiary hospitals and when available is often in poor working conditions and offered in such cumbersome and unresponsive processes that clients do not benefit or choose to seek private care. This is the predominant reason for the large economic burden of medical tourism in Nigeria [13]. Access to emergency care is also very limited. Very few hospitals have facilities and personnel for medical evacuation and when available, the cost excludes most of the population. At the tertiary care level, the main factors responsible for this is poor leadership, poor funding, lack of development of health manpower and consequently, brain drain.

16. PHC as the foundation for health system development

The WHO reform of PHC has as one of its' major thrusts the achievement of UHC via the PHC system and therefore the establishment of PHC as the basis for health system design, development and growth. The misconception and misconstruction of PHC in Nigeria has on the contrary had adverse effect on the system in this regard resulting in stunting of the development of the health system.

Health and social justice: Health as a social good and means to equity and social justice and a responsibility of government: this concept is highly underdeveloped in the psyche of leaders and managers in and beyond the health system and evidenced by the policies and strategies instituted for the system. The misconception of the PHC and persistence on this course despite awareness of its failures and the WHO reformed PHC makes this evident [6]. This is reflected in the fact that public hospital managers are not performance driven and the quality of the services in the facilities do not determine management decisions. Responsiveness to clients is not a core goal of hospital managers. There are no road maps for the development of facilities as there is fundamentally no defined goals and responsibilities of these facilities to the communities they serve. Management goals and priorities are completely at the discretion of the extant manager and there is no obligation to continue good initiatives into succeeding administrations resulting in poor development, waste of resources and entrenchment of the culture of systemic laissez-faire attitude to population health.

The endorsement of the non-professional workforce as competent to deliver care has resulted in a total devaluation of the quality of care in the health system providers and users alike. CHEWS Chemists, nurses, pharmacy shops, fake doctors and all manner of charlatans are allowed to render care. Due to the prohibitive waiting time, direct and opportunity costs of hospital visits, patients seek convenient but unsafe and inappropriate care from these sources resulting in late presentation to the hospitals, increased morbidity and mortality. The misconception and devaluation of quality of care and life has been entrenched to the extent that non-professional health manpower are now licensed to run private health facilities based on standing orders and the task shifting and task sharing strategy [6]. The lack of a quality and data management culture renders this toll on health and life unmeasured and unaccounted for. The government does not take responsibility for this since it is considered good enough for the poor.

Quality management culture: The non-existence of quality management framework in the system has resulted in the stunted development of this all important component of the health system. Quality of Care as a concept and important metric in the structures and processes of care delivery is alien to even the professional health providers. Knowledge and implementation of evidence-based best practice is entirely left to the discretion of individual practitioners without any systemic efforts at evaluation of practice and outcomes. There is a culture of resistance to innovations to implement improvement based on primordial egotistic tendencies [35]. The appropriateness, efficacy, efficiency, and safety of care delivered even in professional settings in tertiary hospitals is often questionable and unaccounted for. There is therefore no framework for responsibility, accountability, development and reformation of the care system towards achieving high-quality care and performance resulting in stunting of development.

Gate keeping and coordination: Unlike the non-professional manpower for the existing PHC, the professional PHC provider in the reformed PHC, has the capacity to provide coordination functions managing gatekeeping to secondary and tertiary care resources. In developed countries this has resulted in more efficient use of health system resources allowing for focusing of high technology care on those most in need of it. Also, secondary care function is mostly integrated with the primary care physicians with most problems being effectively addressed at primary care. The poor capacity for quality care and coordination in the PHCs in Nigeria has resulted in the self-referral of patients to secondary and tertiary care facilities resulting in overcrowding and long waiting times in these facilities and limiting access to care [32]. This in addition to poor funding and equipment of tertiary facilities, contributes to deterring the development of the capacity of these providers for tertiary care. A systemic lack of understanding of these concepts has resulted in confusion of the emerging role of Family Physicians in the Nigerian health system. The terminology primary care in the teaching hospitals where most Family Physicians are trained is irreconcilable with the primary care synonymous with non-professional workforce. Currently there is no coordination of care in the system and consequently patients are receiving very fragmented care with all the attendant adverse impact on quality of care, outcomes, cost and quality of life.

17. Way forward

There is an urgent need to correct these fundamental errors in our health system as the current situation is not only ineffective but constitutes a perpetual journey to poor development.

The time to reform the health system of Nigeria is now more than ever to create a new path to health care access and the desired health outcomes. This will put the country on the right course to a health system that can hope to serve its purpose, build a foundation for development and growth and bring the system in line with the twenty first century.

This reform must be holistic involving all stakeholders: politicians, health manpower including the private sector, general public, community leaders, civil society organizations, global partners and others to ensure buy in, ownership and sustainability. It must include the 4 reform pillars of the WHO reform: leadership and governance, public policies, universal health coverage and service delivery.

Political leadership must own the responsibility for the health of the citizenry and therefore embrace the evidence-based WHO reform agenda. They must engage all stakeholders synergistically in the reform process. However, the capacity of our political leaders as currently constituted to effect this reform is perceived as limited. A major reform to generate the necessary political will to effect the reform can only come from a positive change in the political actors in the country. This will also include major reforms to curb the monumental corruption that exists in the health sector as in other sectors generally in the country. The major critical areas that must be attended to include the PHC policy reform, the urgent holistic restructuring of the health manpower management: increasing the availability and quality of training sites, good work conditions and incentivization of specialization especially for primary care specialists, rural appointments, positive change in the engagement of professional organizations in disputes and high-quality manpower data management.

There is need for development of a primary care movement whose primary goal will be to educate and mobilize all stakeholders to understand the new PHC and drive the momentum to overcome the inertia of political leadership to reform. The movement should be led by health professionals and include civil society organizations, community leaders, the general public, Nigerian health professionals in the diaspora and global actors [2].

The tasks required include:

Education and conscientization of all stakeholders to understand the critical need to build a health system with the capacity to deliver health while creating a foundation for growth and development of the system. A major thrust of critical importance in the process is the reform of the value system of all stakeholders to achieve a prevailing spirit of solidarity, responsibility and accountability without which the nation cannot survive.

Health professional organizations: A multi-faceted engagement is required to achieve a wide range of empowerment covering leadership training, health system organization, dynamics, goals and management, health system regulation, professionalism, interprofessional relationship, team work, data-based management, quality of care, health system advocacy and the PHC reform.

There is need to engage and achieve a renewed commitment to the responsibility for the health of society as a social contract of the professions with society so as to encourage positive change in the sector at all levels. Also, there is need to craft a more functional approach to engagement with the political leadership and mitigate the incessant industrial actions that cripple the system. This will require engagement of the professionals and the political actors to reorient their approach to leadership and management of the system and create a synergy between them. All these are expected to yield dividends in improved interprofessional relations, reduced strike actions, acceptance of innovation, development of quality framework and extension of these into the health professions training.

The Nigerian health professionals in the diaspora have an important role to play as they can share their experiences from developed countries and mentor their home organizations thereby supporting human resources reform which is critical to the strengthening of the system. The health professional bodies can apply a bottom up approach to effect change in the health system from the professionals to the policy makers and catalyze the process of reform. The health professionals as a body have a critical role to play in developing health priorities and designing best practices as in other countries but this is grossly lacking in Nigeria. This has to be corrected and will require actions generated by the professional organizations with commitment to the best interest of the system and advocacy to establish this structure in the health system.

18. Research and innovation

The health professionals need to reform the existing poor ethical research culture. Research and evidence-based innovation in the system cannot happen without this. The support of government and donors is very important in this regard but requires the reform of research culture. All areas are important but system-based practice, quality of care and outcomes are needed urgently to generate evidence to guide system development and practice. This will increase the culture of innovation and its acceptance and improve ownership, quality of services and efficiency of the system.

Regulatory Framework: There is a critical need to develop and entrench a strong effective regulatory framework in the system. There is generally poor culture of regulation in the country but the consequence in the health sector is grievous. The system cannot achieve its goal without an effective regulatory framework as obtains in developed countries. The health professionals and their organizations have a critical role to play here and must champion this cause. Continuing professional development, renewal of licencing, reaccreditations through credible processes, periodic relicensing examinations, etc., are critically important in ensuring that professionals and facilities are up to date to assure technical quality of care. The proliferation of charlatan practices needs to be curbed. The practice of consultations, prescriptions and dispensing of drugs from all manner of sources needs to be regulated to curb the level of unsafe, poor-quality care abundant in the system.

Global Partners: Donors should channel donations and aid less to vertical programmes embedded in the old PHC and channel it to structures and processes that support the development of the reformed PHC and health insurance coverage as done by health fund in Sokoto state. Also, they can create incentives to retain health workers in Nigeria especially rural areas to support the reform process. There is need for the global community to take measures to address trans-border migration of health workers especially from poor resource countries to high resource nations in the interest of global health equity. Donations and aids to poor nations cannot translate to desired cost-effective health outcomes if the critical input of health professionals required for success is unavailable. The training of health professionals in Nigerian public universities has hitherto been almost entirely borne by the government and the brain drain represents not just a flight of human capital but of developmental resources used in their training and the consequent impoverishment of our health system.

19. Health human resources management

The most critical input in any system is the human resources and the failure of the current PHC system has clearly demonstrated this. The challenge of health human resources development in Nigeria is indeed daunting, given the current state of socioeconomic, political, security and health system contexts. However, this challenge must be addressed to stop further waste of resources and retrogression of the health system and the country.

The reformed PHC requires that primary care be delivered by specialist primary care physicians especially family physicians and other health professionals working in teams with the populations empanelled to those teams.

The challenge of manpower management requires a positive change in government's sense of responsibility and investments for all sectors especially the education and health sectors to improve quality and quantity of training. Manpower employment and retention requires that government must change its' contentious posture that mismanages industrial disputes in the health and education sectors. There must be a synergy between government and health professionals as allies in constructive engagements in design, regulation and management of the health system and in particular to address issues relating to work conditions for health manpower. The existing number of physicians (and all other health professionals) is abysmally poor and cannot meet the required placements. A creative and committed roadmap must be drawn as fundamental to the reform plan on how to efficiently deploy available manpower in the short term and extend same in the future. Majority of the physicians in the country are not specialized. The National Post Graduate Medical College of Nigeria has a diplomate program in Family Medicine which can be harnessed to increase the number of physicians trained to deliver care in the context of primary care ensuring that all physicians in the primary care space are better prepared to offer quality first-contact care. This would then facilitate their deployment in empanelled systems as would be designed to directly offer care, supervise and support care teams and increase available sites for training of house officers who would also be integrated into the scheme. Also, at undergraduate level, family medicine training should be mandated in all medical schools to ensure that all graduates are prepared for primary care on graduation. This approach has worked very well in a LMIC like Cuba [36].

20. System reconstruction

The national health insurance scheme offers a mechanism for transforming the health system and implementing the reform of the PHC. Currently the NHIS and the PHC system under the NPHCDA are the two health delivery pathways in the system. The new NHIA Act that makes health insurance compulsory in Nigeria demands that the service delivery must extend to everywhere and everyone mandating universal access to health and thereby mandating only one delivery system. The critical issue then is how to create a system that is capable of achieving this mandate by aligning structures and processes to the goal. The WHO PHC reform provides the pathway to achieve this by organizing the NHIS on the reformed PHC model. The resource limitations in deploying the remodelling across the entire system is obvious. The proposal here is therefore to create a road map wherein the remodelling can start where resources permit and extend to others over time so as to commit the system in the right direction to development and growth.

21. NHIS

The NHIS coverage in urban areas suffers the challenge of quality and efficiency more than availability of facilities and personnel unlike in rural areas. The reform should be to reorganize the delivery system to achieve empanelment, physician led primary care approach offering, comprehensive, continuing, coordinated, person-centered quality care. This would involve professionals training in family medicine, quality of care, quality management system and regulation of all practices including public and private. The quality and responsiveness of services need to be improved especially, timeliness to remove the barrier of long waiting time and improvement in patient information access.

The role of the private sector is critically important as they control a significant proportion of the service delivery system and must be properly harnessed into the system. Lessons can be learned from the British system where the primary care is delivered entirely by private providers under regulation from the quality systems of the NHS [26].

Empanelment requires the mapping of the population into segments to be served by defined health teams. The existing ward health system has already mapped the population and defined teams of nurses and CHEWs to cater for them. These teams should be further developed and empanelled to defined providers to incorporate them into the NHIS delivery system. This therefore requires that all PHC services covering vertical programs should be mainstreamed into the NHIS services and duplicate funding redeployed to other needs.

The NHIS program available for rural dwellers is the community-based scheme which has so far not gained much traction due to the lack of government support, strong community health development committees, ignorance, poverty and also lack of functional health facilities. Rebuilding of dilapidated facilities, government subsidization of CBI and mobilization of community awareness will increase ownership of community-based insurance scheme and utilization of the PHC facilities in rural areas. This will also be facilitated by the implementation of the VGSHIP reducing the burden of indigent people in the communities. The shortage of professional health manpower can be mitigated by incentivizing rural posting of doctors and other professionals and use of telehealth and other adaptations of information technology to provide clinical care and supervisory support to the existing non-professional manpower in empanelled teams. Where unhindered by security considerations, incentivized rural exchanges for urban-based professionals could also alleviate the shortage.

The NHIS coverage for the informal sector needs to be deepened by government subsidy, increasing awareness and enrolment of the population in this bracket as done in other developing countries like India and Chile [2].

These steps would set the reform into motion harnessing the available resources to achieve efficiently, both geographical and quality access to those in areas that can be covered now and set a template for growth to cover other areas in the future. A commitment to the road map for development of the system is necessary ensuring that system growth is sustained from one political administration to the next. The NHIA should therefore be conscientized and empowered to perform their role in ensuring the health of the population by taking charge of all health service delivery driven by a quality management culture and responsiveness. Regulatory authorities must be built into the new system structure to regularly set standards, monitor performance, regulate compliance, research system dynamics and performance and provide guidance as done in developed countries [26].

Leadership and Governance: reform in this domain requires whole country effort to reduce the level of corruption and irresponsible leadership that permeates and destroys the whole system. As regards the health system, reconstruction of the system should include streamlining the structures for funding, financing and purchasing of health services into structures that are transparent and aligned to performance and goal achievement. The current system is so convoluted and opaque that funds and its deployment cannot be tracked. The essential package of health services needs to be upgraded and reformed to correspond to basic health plans of the NHIS which is the minimum required to offer a health coverage. The reformed EPHS should therefore be the basis for determining the health budget in order to create appropriate alignments of goals, budget and delivery structures and processes.

The government must raise health budgets to meet the recommendations of at least 15% of national budget

The NPHCDA services should be mainstreamed into the basic health plans of the NHIS and therefore the funds for RMNCAH services should be mainstreamed into the NHIS via the state health insurance authorities. All donations and grants for these should be tracked through the NHIS ensuring delivery of services and shifting of funds from BHPs to deepen coverage of other services where BHP offers duplication of RMNCAH services.

The statutory domiciliation of governance of PHC under the local government authorities needs to be changed as this level of government has not been allowed to function and so is incapable of managing PHC. Again, even if they were to be strengthened, the responsibility for the successful funding and management of a professional led reformed PHC is beyond the capacity of a local government authority. The current legislation on health as a responsibility of the three tiers of government therefore needs to be amended in line with the realities and for ensuring a successful health system. The state health insurance authorities should be in charge of the NHIS services deployed through a reformed PHC model.

Conclusion: In Nigeria, access to health care in all its dimensions as a function of structure and function of the health system and its interaction with people is very poor.

Poor leadership perpetuated the misconception of Primary health care and stunted the development of the health system.

New paths to improvement require system reconstruction and a reform of the primary health care system now more than ever.

Conflict of interest

The author declares no conflict of interest.

Author details

Vivien O. Abah
Department of Family Medicine, University of Benin Teaching Hospital, Benin City, Edo State, Nigeria

*Address all correspondence to: vienabah@gmial.com

References

[1] World Health Organization. Universal Health Coverage. Available at http://www.who.int [Accessed August 29, 2022]

[2] World Health Organization. Primary Health Care. Now More Than Ever. WorldHealthReport2008. Available at http://www.who.int [Accessed June 23 2012]

[3] Cu A, Meister S, Lefebvre B, Ridde V. Assessing healthcare access using the Levesque's conceptual framework–a scoping review. International Journal for Equity in Health. 7 May 2021;**20**(1):116. DOI: 10.1186/s12939-021-01416-3. PMID:33962627; PMCID:PMC8103766

[4] Adedini SA, Odimegwu C, Bamiwuye O, Fadeyibi O, Wet N. Barriers to accessing health care in Nigeria: Implication for child survival. Global Health Action. 14 Mar 2014;7:23499. DOI: 10.3402/gha.v.7.23499

[5] Nigerian Population. 2022

[6] Federal Government of Nigeria. National Strategic Health Development Plan II (2018-2022). Available at https://ngfrepository.org.ng [Accessed September 22, 2021]

[7] Amata D. Budget: N3,453 per Capita for the medical care of Every Nigerian in 2022. 2022. Available at https://www.dataphyte.com [Accessed August 8, 2022]

[8] Nigeria- World Bank Data. 2022 [Accessed August 28, 22]

[9] Number of Doctors in Nigeria from 2017 to 2019. Available at www.statista .com

[10] National Primary Health Care Development Agency. Minimum Standards for Primary Health Care in Nigeria. Available at https://ngfrepository.org.ng [Accessed September 10, 21]

[11] Christian Aid. Assessment of Primary Health Centres in selected States of Nigeria. E: nigeria-info@christian-aid.org, www.christianaid.org.uk/Nigeria

[12] Federal Republic of Nigeria. National Health Act 2014. Available at https://nigeriahealthwatch.com [Accessed August 25, 22]

[13] Adeyemi S. Nigeria Set to become Destination for Medical Tourism, Reverse Brain Drain-Minister. 2022. Available at www. fmic.gov.ng [Accessed August 25, 22]

[14] National Primary Health Care Development Agency. Integrating Primary Health Care Governance in Nigeria. Available at https://ngfrepository.org.ng [Accessed August 19, 22]

[15] Murray CJL, Frenk J. A framework for assessing the performance of health systems. Bulletin of the World Health Organization. 2000;**78**(6):717-731

[16] Guidelines for Administration, Disbursement, Monitoring and Fund management for Basic Health Care Provision Fund. 2016. Available at https://www.health.gov.ng [Accessed April 25, 20]

[17] WHO. Essential health Packages: What are they for? What do they Change? Draft Technical Brief No. 2. 2008. WHO Available at http://www.who.int [Accessed September 25, 2021]

[18] The Essential Health Service Package in Nigeria. Tropical Health Matters. 2018. Available at https://www.hfgproject.org/essential-package-of-health-services-country-snapshotnigeria/ [Accessed June 5, 2021]

[19] The World Bank. Deep Structural Reforms Guided by Evidence Are urgently Needed to Lift Millions of Nigerians out of Poverty, Says New World Bank Report. Press Release No. 2022/052/AFW March 22, 2022

[20] Popoola N. 22 years after, NHIS suffer slow patronage amid complaints, corruption others. Available at www.punchng.com [Accessed August 4, 22]

[21] National Health Insurance Authority-Act-2022. 2022. Available at https:// nhis.gov.ng [Accessed August 4, 22]

[22] Ismaila Chafe Health Insurance. Vulnerable Group Fund to cater for 83 m Nigerians. 2022. PM NEWS. Available at www.pmnewsnigeria.com [Accessed August 4, 22]

[23] Biriowo K. FG disbuses N56bn Basic Healthcare Provision Funds to 36 States, FCT. Tribune Online. African Newspapers of Nigeria PLC. 2022. Available at www.tribunronlineng.com [Accessed August 19, 22]

[24] Dutta A, Hongoro C. Scaling Up National Health Insurance in Nigeria: Learning from Case Studies of India, Colombia, and Thailand. Washington, DC: Futures Group, Health Policy Project; 2013

[25] The Primary Health Care Performance Initiative. The PHCPI conceptual Framework. Available at www.improvingphc.org [Accessed August 5, 22]

[26] Tikkanen R, Osborn R, Mossialos E, Djordjevic A, Wharton GA. International Health Care System Profiles: England. 2020

[27] Uzochukwu BSC. Primary Health Care Systems (PRIMASYS): Case study from Nigeria. World Health Organization alliancehpsr@who.int http://www.who.int/alliance-hpsr

[28] Adeloye D, David AR, Olaogun AA, Auta A, Adesokan A, Gadanya M, et al. Health workforce and governance: The crisis in Nigeria. Human Resources for Health. 2017;**15**:32

[29] Adebayo A, Akinyemi OO. What are you really doing in this Country?: Emigration Intentions of Nigerian Doctors and their Policy Implications for Human Resource for Health Management. Journal of International Migration and Integration. 2021. DOI: 10.1007/s12134-021-00898-y

[30] WHO. Low Quality Health Care is increasing the burden of illness and health costs globally. 2018. Available at http://www.who.int/servicedeliverysafety/quality-report/en/ [Accessed April 3, 2017]

[31] Uchejeso OMI, Etukudoh NS, Chongs ME, Ime DM. Challenges of Inter-Professional Teamwork in Nigerian Healthcare

[32] Koce F, Randhawa G, Ochieng B. Understanding healthcare self-referral in Nigeria from the service user's perspective: A qualitative study of Niger State. BMC Health Service Research. 2019;**19**:209

[33] Ogunfowokan O, Mora M. Time expectation and satisfaction: Patient's experience at National Hospital Abuja, Nigeria. Afr j Prm Health Care. Family Medicine. 2012;**4**(1):a398-a404. DOI: 10.4102/phcfm.v4i1.398

[34] Ogaji DS, Mezie- Okoye MM. Waiting Time and Patient Satisfaction: Survey of Patients Seeking Care at the General Outpatient Clinic of University of Port Harcourt Teaching Hospital Port Harcourt. Medicine Journal. 2017;**11**:148-155

[35] Asakitikpi AE. Healthcare Coverage and Affordability in Nigeria: An Alternative Model to Equitable Healthcare Delivery

[36] Suarez IRM, Sacasas JAF, Garcia FD. Cuban medical education: Aiming for the Six-Star Doctor. MEDICC Review. 2008;**10**:4

Chapter 9

Home Visitation by Community Health Workers

Hilda Kawaya

Abstract

Community health workers are faced with challenges in the community during home visits. The re-engineering of primary health care services in South Africa brought a new cadre of community health workers that relieved the extra workload of primary health care nurses of conducting home visits as one of the activities. The findings of the study conducted in the Tshwane District culminated in the challenges of community, logistical, occupational, human resource, and managerial in nature. The CHWs stated the need for respect and acceptance by the community during home visits, improved planning related to delegation of households by Outreach Leaders and provision of material resources, and the support by managers for career development through training and education for various disease prevention. This indicated that the training of community health workers needs to be formalized and in-service education related to home visits should be planned, structured, and supported by the Department of Health.

Keywords: challenges, perceived, community health workers, home visit, primary health care

1. Introduction

This chapter defines home visits, community health worker and primary health care, the overview of home visits, the purpose of home visits, the historical perspective of home visits, the process of home visits, the advantages and disadvantages of home visits, challenges encountered by community health workers (CHWs) during home visits from a South African perspective, and report from the study done in 2020 by CHWs in the Tshwane district.

2. Definition of home visits

A home visit is a formal interaction between a nurse and an individual's place of residence designed to provide nursing care related to the identified need.

3. Definition of community health worker

Community health worker means an individual with an in-depth understanding of the community culture and language, who has received standardized job-related training, which is of shorter duration than health professionals, and whose the primary goal is to provide culturally appropriate health services to the community. CHW is an individual employed by the state, allocated at a PHC facility by a nongovernmental entity, and receives a stipend for the services rendered in the community.

4. Primary health care

Primary health care is health care based on scientifically evidence-based care by socially acceptable standards, which is universally accessible to individuals and their families at a cost the community and the country can afford by being self-reliant and by self-determination. PHC is rendered to individuals and families who are residents of the area surrounding the community clinic by health workers.

5. Overview of home visits

Families and individuals visit the primary health care (PHC) clinic daily and/or monthly to be assessed for acute and chronic ailments as well as monitor compliance. Noncompliance to treatment will warrant that the community health worker (CHW) visits the individual more frequently to establish the reasons for clinic nonattendance and noncompliance to treatment regimens [1]. CHW programs are designed to target hard-to-reach communities that are more than 5 km from a health facility or in the lowest socioeconomic areas [2]. The PHC clinics provide preventive, promotive, curative, and rehabilitative services to the community within a 5-km radius. Currently, the clinics consult with the ward-based outreach teams to allocate CHWs to do home visits to individuals who default on treatment and are noncompliant with treatment. CHWs are responsible for home visits to make sure that vulnerable groups are getting adequate care and are not missed in the health system. CHWs are currently paid stipends by the Department of Health and through nongovernmental organizations [3].

Currently, an estimated 5482 PHC outreach teams are caring for the uninsured population of South Africa, and the teams are required to reach 84% of the total population who are based in rural areas, informal urban settlements, and townships [4]. In the financial year 2014/2015, it was estimated that there were 86 teams in Tshwane covering 46 wards, with 39 trained team leaders and 217 CHWs [5]. The services are available, accessible, and affordable [6], and are provided at homes, schools, and other public and private institutions because health care is a right for all citizens. The role of the CHWs among others is to do home visits [7]. Home visit services originated in Great Britain, dating back to the 1850s, and focused on improving health and hygiene in families with young children. The families were visited for the continuation of nursing care and support. According to the study [8], home visits offer a viable strategy to avoid challenges associated with obtaining health from clinics, which include difficulty in scheduling clinic appointments, long waiting lines, and expensive transport.

The evaluation of the effectiveness of the home-visit program for high-risk pregnant women [9] found that at least one visitation during pregnancy was effective in preventing preterm births. Participating in the home-visit program reduced the risk of adverse outcomes in a disadvantaged population [10]. It was found that home visits are part of larger programs that might have positive effects on individuals, including exercise programs, improved assessment methods by medical professionals, or fall prevention [11]. Skilled health workers do home visits, but in areas where there is a lack of health providers, trained community members, called CHWs, are used instead. These workers are trained to perform basic preventative and curative care and to assist families in seeking necessary care at a healthcare facility.

The role of CHWs in Lesotho dates to 1979 when the country embraced primary health care (PHC) and improved the efforts to reach underserved and remote areas [12]. The CHWs' scope ranges from core roles of disease prevention, early detection of ill-health, community advocacy, outreach services, and assisting in accessing services through referrals and home visits. The CHWs understand their roles and responsibilities regarding health promotion. However, the changes in disease burden have resulted in a shift in roles and this is affecting their health promotion practice and experience. You et el. [13] reported that the outcomes of health workers doing home visits for at-risk mothers in the United States are less effective compared to nurses, who are better suited to enhance and determine physical and psychological health, and decrease the use of emergency medical services. Bheekie and Bradley [14] reported that home visiting has been demonstrated as being effective when mounted by professionals, but low and middle-income countries (LMICs), such as South Africa, cannot afford nurses and will not be able to train the personnel necessary to render such support until at least by the year 2050.

In 2010, the South African National Department of Health (NDoH) launched a national PHC initiative to strengthen health promotion, disease prevention, and early disease detection called reengineering of primary health care (rPHC) to provide preventive and health-promoting community-based PHC model [15]. A key component of rPHC is the use of ward-based outreach teams (WBOTS) staffed by generalist CHWs to do home visits and provide care to families and communities [16, 17]. CHWs are a core in the community-based PHC model and the complex contextual challenges they face during home visits and the development of skills in community care need specific attention [18]. Health facilities are challenged by limited staffing, resources, infrastructure, and access to PHC clinics is affected by distance, financial constraints, and transport availability.

6. The purpose of home visits

The purpose of the home visit is to have face-to-face contact at an individual's home, with a healthcare professional. The home visit allows an assessment of the home environment and family situation to provide for healthcare-related activities. It is done to reduce the defaulter rate and to enhance compliance with treatment [7]. Home visits provide opportunities for professional development, as well as improve the life orientation skills of healthcare students [19].

7. Historical perspective

Globally, home visits were intended to improve health and hygiene in families with young children [7]. A home visit is vital to reducing maternal and infant morbidity and mortality [20]. A healthcare project in Egypt recommended four home visits to women and their infants during the postnatal period within 24 h of delivery, on day 4 after birth, on day 7 after birth, and a clinical visit on day 40 [21]. American Indian and Alaska Native people have used informal home visits as a traditional cultural practice to take care of and address the needs of young children and families and improved outcomes in these areas [22].

Salami and Brieger [23] stated that the benefits of home visits by trained community health workers can change newborn practices. Rotheram-Borus et al. [8] confirmed that at least one visitation during pregnancy would reduce the risk of preterm births. Health workers during their home visits were able to keep track of non-facility-based births, which were not recorded officially and affected the calculations of infant mortality [24]. Trainees in medicine can gain experience and confidence in making house calls by doing structured home visits [25]. The focus of home visits expanded to other areas such as care of the elderly. The authors further reported that home visits are proposed to be an essential component of general practice care in the provision of comprehensive person-centered care for the elderly.

Home visits are an integral part of primary care provided by family physicians and medical assistants to homebound elderly individuals living in private households, and not by communities [26]. Preventative home visits may have a positive effect on healthcare costs by decreasing nursing home admission, hospitalizations, and the length of stay in hospitals [27]. Home visiting services are part of the national health systems in most countries in Western Europe, where services are voluntary and free to all families [7].

The role of professional nurses' in home visits as stated by Grant et al. [17] reported that health facilities faced the challenge of limited staffing and resources. The shortage of nurses at PHC clinics made their role to conduct home visits compromised. Wells et al. [28] agreed that, to prevent diseases and promote health, the role of community nurses was to conduct home visits irrespective of work overload. However, it is important to recognize that the clinical proficiency of the nurse performing the home visits had a heavy influence on visits due to their experience, which assists them to diagnose challenges and refer to relevant healthcare providers [29].

In the study by Bheekie and Bradley [14], the establishment of district management teams (DMT) to improve the primary health system increases life expectancy, decreases child and maternal mortality, combats HIV and AIDS, and decreases the tuberculosis burden. The effective use of CHWs is by allocating them to 250 families each, to address health problems. The PHC outreach team consists of a professional nurse, an environmental officer, a health promoter, and six CHWs in a municipal ward who work together with the designated nurses at the clinic to provide comprehensive care to this population, from health promotion to the treatment of minor ailments [30]. According to Kane et al. [31], more than five million CHWs are active globally and are known for their effectiveness and importance in providing services to communities [32]. CHWs are trained government workers allocated at facilities and the community recognizes them as health professionals and an extension of the formal health system.

Kok et al. [33] stated that CHWs had their origins in China in the 1920s and were precursors to the "barefoot doctors" movement in the 1950s, they indicated that CHWs' are groups of health workers who work outside health facilities directly with people in their homes, neighborhoods, communities, and other nonclinical spaces where health and diseases are produced. Zulliger et al. [34] regarded CHWs as health workers conducting functions related to health care delivery; trained in some way in the context of the intervention and having no formal professional or paraprofessional certificate or degree in tertiary education. The role of CHWs is to conduct household profiling, screening, and health education through supervision by the professional nurse team leader [29]. In South Africa, CHWs are expected to assess health needs;

facilitate service access; provide community-based information, education, and psychosocial support; deliver basic health care; and support community campaigns [35]. PHC training package identifies 12 roles that are to be performed by the CHWs working in PHC, which are home-based care, counseling, support and stress relief, health promotion and education at a household level, referral to relevant departments, initiative and support home-based projects, liaison between NDoH and the community, mobilization against diseases and poor health through campaigns, Directly Supervised Treatment Support (DOTS), screening of health-related clinic cards for compliance or default, assessment of health status for all family members and giving advice, weighing infants and babies and recording in "Road to Health" card, and providing prevention of mother-to-child transmission of HIV/AIDS [4].

Kelly et al. [36] reported that the NDoH was developing a policy framework to regulate the role of CHWs and their working conditions and further asserts that shifting tasks and care responsibilities from professionals is necessary to meet the needs of the health care service. CHWs are trained to accompany HIV individuals on ART and do routine home visits to monitor side effects and appointment reminders [37]. The role of CHWs is to collaborate with community leaders in providing basic health and environmental service in rural areas, create a link between the facility and the community, and are paid salaries by the Ministry of Health [38]. In the paper by Ref [39], the role of CHWs in countries has contributed to better outcomes; however, in South Africa, the health outcomes are suboptimal in areas of maternal and child health. Home visits by CHWs during pregnancy can play a role in improving thermal care, early and exclusive breastfeeding, and hygienic cord care practices in different settings [22].

At the international conference on primary health care at Alma-Ata in 1978 where a declaration of "Health for All" by the year 2000 was made by the representatives, CHWs' role in providing PHC was highlighted [32]. The World Health Organization (WHO) has identified five key elements to achieving this goal: reducing exclusion and social disparities in health (universal coverage reforms); principles of equity, access, empowerment, community self-determination, and inter-sectoral collaboration. Universal health coverage (UHC) is aspired by most countries in terms of rights to health care, financial protection, and utilization of healthcare services on an equitable basis. UHC indicates equity of access and financial risk protection [40] and community care is a crucial contribution that is affordable with running costs of less than one dollar per capita per year [41]. The recent Astana Declaration (2018) has emphasized the critical role of PHC in advancing UHC. The potential contribution of CHWs to supporting UHC is commendable [42].

UHC, broadly, means that all people receive the health services they need, including health initiatives designed to promote better health, prevent illness, and provide treatment, rehabilitation, and palliative care of sufficient quality to be effective while at the same time ensuring that the use of these services does not expose the individual to financial hardship. The District Health System (DHS) in South Africa provides an equitable, efficient, and effective health system based on the principles of the PHC approach. The National Health Insurance (NHI) systems and the DHS model are key elements of UHC in South Africa. The DHS depicts a set of activities such as community involvement, integrated and holistic healthcare delivery, intersectoral collaboration, and a strong "bottom-up" approach to planning, policy development, and management. NHI aims to provide funds that will improve access to health services for all South Africans [43] and to rectify the public-private funding inequality. NHI includes rPHC, which focuses on the prevention of diseases, including three streams of municipal ward-based PHC outreach teams, school health teams, and district-based clinical specialist teams [29]. In terms of cost, a preliminary policy paper issued by the government estimated that NHI will cost R255 billion per year by 2025 if implemented as planned over 15 years [44]. To achieve the principles of PHC, together with inclusion in the NHI and UHC, the employment of CHWs commenced.

The health services in which CHWs work often present preconditions or limitations to function [33]. The challenges found in the study of CHWs in Lesotho are demotivation because of inconsistent incentives, lack of supplies, community attitude, increased workload, gaps in training, and lack of standardized reporting tools [11]. CHWs work in an environment where trust and confidentiality play a cornerstone in social relationships. CHWs interact with other family members during home visits and discussing confidential information seemed to be challenging if family members were present and could lead to unwanted disclosure of sensitive information [17]. Families failed to obtain medications due to transportation and financial problems [29]. Transport is identified as a challenge in the study of workers in Malawi [38]. Management apathy around allowances for CHWs in Kenya is a source of feelings of devaluation and of not having control over one's work sphere [31].

Other barriers included the lack of career prospects for CHWs, lack of formal recognition as government employees of the health system (even though the stipend is paid through the government pay system), low incentives, and delayed payments [45]. CHWs preferred better financial recognition for their work, an increase in stipend, and proof of their work for prospects, raincoats, Christmas hampers, and tokens to help mitigate financial constraints [46]. The CHWs mentioned their role in solving social issues in the community, but the stipend did not match the extra work they did on top of health issues. Working in the community allows opportunities to channel their values and beliefs into concrete actions with opportunities for self-actualization [31]. A perceived lack of personal safety was found to affect motivation to work at locations and into people resigning. Young female health workers felt unsafe, scared of substance abuse among young men, violent assaults, verbal abuse, accusations, and were afraid of contracting infections [22].

Climate, environmental challenges, and the need to cover large distances hampered CHWs' performance of their duties. It was reported that the CHWs' had difficulties in reaching communities because of flooding [33]. A study done in Uganda for the visitation of mothers during prenatal and postnatal by Village Health Teams proved that the teams could not navigate large geographical areas in some cases and had low incentives for Village Health Teams to travel long distances [47]. Traditionally in Jordan, women are not supposed to leave the house for 40 days post-delivery, mothers preferred that the home visit should be conducted by a female CHW in the presence of a family member to enhance a sense of security [19].

8. Advantages of home visits

The advantages of home visits are ranging from and not conclusive to the following:

- It provides an assessment window into the household characteristics.
- The nurse obtains the full picture of the home environment the individuals reside in.

- Identification of the influence of the environment on the individual's health.
- It allows the CHW to view the individuals' relationship with family members and the community.
- It is an opportunity for a CHW to view the individual's performance of activities of daily living.
- It gives the CHW a perspective to plan and evaluate interventions in a natural setting.
- It allows a CHW to recognize unidentified health and social needs.

9. Disadvantages of home visits

There are a few disadvantages of home visits as stated below:

- A stigma attached to the family's self-perspective of incompetence.
- It is not cost-effective for a health worker to travel to one individual and see them at home unlike seeing them at the clinic and achieving the goal of consulting twenty individuals in a day.

10. The process of home visits, a home visitation program

The home visitation program in South Africa is structured by the outreach team leaders who allocate different individuals to a specific CHW to visit the homes in a particular month. The nursing process approach of assessment, diagnosing, planning, implementation, evaluation documentation, and termination is utilized by following the outlined steps to explain the program [48].

10.1 Step 1

Initiation of the home visit whereby the CHW introduces themself to establish rapport.

10.2 Step 2

Conduct a preliminary assessment by reviewing the individual's history and documentation to determine the health care needs related to biological, psychological, environmental, sociocultural, behavioral, and health system determinants of health.

10.3 Step 3

Formulate a diagnosis based on the assessment.

10.4 Step 4

Plan to review the previous interventions made and their results. Prioritize the needs and identify those that need immediate attention. Develop goals and objectives for the visit and determine the levels of care involved. Consider the individual's circumstances and consent related to the visit and time of visits. Identify appropriate interventions to address problems. Mobilize resources, supplies, and equipment. Plan for evaluation of the home visit.

10.5 Step 5

Implementation of the plans made by priority and dealing with any distractions.

10.6 Step 6

Evaluate the response to the interventions, short-term and long-term outcomes, the quality of planning and implementation of the home visit, and the quality of care.

10.7 Step 7

Document the individuals' assessment, interventions, individuals' responses to care, outcomes of interventions, plans of care, and the individual's health status at discharge.

10.8 Step 8

Plan for termination on the first visit, inform the individual about the number of visits and their duration, review the goals and objectives, and make referrals where necessary.

11. Challenges encountered by community health workers

Below are narrative perspectives of community health workers from the study done by the author.

11.1 Community challenges

Community challenges emerged as the first perceived challenge by the CHWs. Various challenges from the community posed a problem in accessing the community members during home visits. This included community access, animosity, mistrust, noncompliance to treatment, nonrecognition, acceptance, and public environmental health.

11.1.1 Community access

The CHWs were faced with difficulty in accessing members of the community during the day and the attitude they received from community members hampered access. CHWs reported that when going to visit individuals at homes, they meet people in the street calling them names and swearing at them and when they reach the designated homes individuals will chase them away or send dogs after them. The CHWs are required to map 250 household registrations as part of the workload for the area that is allocated to them. All the households should be captured and followed up to reach all members of the designated community linked to the PHC clinic.

11.1.2 Community animosity and mistrust

CHWs mentioned that data capturing included registration of the water meter reading, which led to the community members asking questions about the relation of meter checking to health and illness. CHWs were faced with mistrust and resentment from the community due to the belief that their roles were not in support of community needs. The lack of respect from the community has been seen to demotivate CHWs [45].

Several factors undermining the work of CHWs, as stated in the study by Mhlongo and Lutge [32], were different perceptions of the CHW roles, lack of knowledge and skills, and lack of stakeholders and community support.

11.1.3 Community noncompliance with treatment

Individuals with chronic conditions, TB, and HIV default to treatment and are not compliant with taking the medication. Follow-up is done to monitor compliance with treatment. Home visits are conducted to follow up with defaulters of treatment and to encourage compliance with treatment. The individuals are traced back to their addresses to keep them on track with and to comply with the treatment prescribed.

11.1.4 Nonrecognition and acceptance by the community

The CHWs reported that the clinic does not provide uniforms but only name tags. The uniform that they wear was provided by the NGO before being transferred to the clinics. The lack of uniform and name tags make the community not recognize and accept the workers as professionals and they are given a bad attitude. In the study about the role of CHWs [46], it was reported that the workers asked for "branded" goods, such as t-shirts, hats, or ID cards, to identify them as part of the health team. The provision of branded goods would prevent them from being viewed with suspicion by the community.

11.1.5 Public environmental health

The CHWs assist with the cleaning of the home, such as dirty windows, and open windows for fresh air before commencing with procedures. The unsafe and unkempt environment in the community leads to CHWs to extend their scope of work by cleaning the household and referring the challenges to the social development ministry.

11.2 Logistical challenges

The government should devise a means of providing the CHW programs with transport and absorb them to be permanent employees with all benefits. CHW programs tend to be unsustainable at scale when there is poor planning, vague and/or extensive CHW scopes of work, lack of community and health system buy-in, resource scarcity, inadequate training, low incentives to the CHWs, and poor supervision [45].

11.2.1 Ineffective planning and delegation

The concept of walking the distance from house to house and to and from the clinic to report and clock out poses a challenge even though it is structured daily. The CHW program should be planned so that CHWs report weekly to the OTLs at a designated area in the clinic. The CHW should draw a monthly schedule and submit it to the manager for approval.

11.2.2 Lack of transport

The CHWs walk distances to individuals' homes after they have reported at the clinic and at the end of the home visit go back to the clinic to clock out. The clinic does not provide transport for CHWs. They are not allowed in government vehicles as they do not have indemnity. Weather conditions and the fact that the CHWs are contract workers also mitigate the challenge of transport. CHWs in other areas did not access formal modes of transport and instead walked to and from their allocated area of work.

11.3 Occupational challenges

The scope of practice of CHWs does not include aspects of mental health and domestic abuse and cannot intervene when faced with situations. The CHWs refer the matters beyond their control to the police and social workers because it is not covered in their training.

11.3.1 Exposure to ethical-legal risks

The CHWs gave information about this insufficient training, which causes distress when dealing with individuals. Other health topics were not covered in their training, which made them frustrated. The insufficient training given to CHWs will lead them to be involved in legal cases and can be found to have violated ethical issues.

11.3.2 Exposure to psychological risks

The CHWs have trouble dealing with emotions and would be brave in front of individuals not to expose their sadness in seeing children with terminal conditions. They cry privately when they reach their homes. They pray daily not to meet dangerous individuals in the community. The CHWs experience emotional stress of coping with difficult circumstances of being scared to venture into the community. Exposure to sick individuals causes emotional distress and frustration.

11.3.3 Exposure to safety risks in the community

The CHWs mentioned that the nurses at the clinic will give referrals to trace individuals who defaulted treatment of TB, others are XDR or MDR individuals, and end up being exposed to health risks of contracting diseases because of insufficient information given to them about the individual status.

The lack of face masks when visiting homes can lead to workers contracting airborne diseases. There were concerns about CHW's safety, identification, debriefing, and risk of contracting diseases [29].

11.3.4 Insufficient equipment and resources

The CHWs reported challenges of limited resources of having to carry blood pressure machines to different homes on certain days. Lack of data on cell phones to call the OTLs or to summon the ambulance when faced with emergencies during home visits. The cell phones issued had a short lifespan. The lack of material resources creates a challenge and financial burden for community workers, which can lead to feelings of frustration and spending their own money to counter the limited resources [47].

11.3.5 Working relationship problems with clinic staff

The lack of medical aid to consult when ill poses a challenge to CHWs and this is seen by the clinic staff, making CHWs queue like any other individual visiting the facility.

The lack of support from clinic staff leads to stress and frustration [29]. Managers reported that the CHW's workload was very heavy and their working conditions are difficult and mentioned the lack of space, stationery, and equipment.

11.4 Human resources challenges

The human resource department in the clinics does not include CHWs in the skill professional development plan. The CHWs reported no opportunities to improve their skills and see growth in their chosen job and the reluctance of the clinic to include them during in-service training.

11.4.1 Inadequate opportunities for personal development and promotion

The CHWs have no opportunities for promotion from one level to the other, they remain in one category. There should be a growth pathway for CHWs to ensure that the persons with experience can achieve higher levels of employment and mentor the newer applicants in the program [4]. In South Africa, the Human Resource for Health Strategy estimated that the critical need gap persists with a shortage of over three thousand formally qualified CHWs and over two thousand qualified home-based caregivers [45].

11.4.2 Inadequate training and education

The CHWs reported that there is inadequate training when they observed that other CHWs were performing the same skill differently. Peer training is encouraged in areas that were not covered in the CHW course. Conducting more in-service education will make sure that the acquired skills and knowledge are not lost forever [37]. Formalization of CHWs' training about procedures done during home visits will bring job satisfaction. It was recommended that the training of the CHWs should be incorporated into the Expanded Public Works Programme (EPWP) training strategy, which will enable the CHWs to obtain a formal qualification that is aligned with national standards [4]. The general training of CHWs as generalist health workers is ideal, but program-specific training is effective and ensures that core knowledge and skills are effectively relayed [49].

11.4.3 Unconducive conditions of service

The CHWS sign a contract every year and they have been in the temporary position for more than five years. The CHWs expressed anger and frustration when narrating the aspect of stipends and signing contracts of employment every year. The gifts received from employers helped mitigate financial requests [46]. CHWs reflected negatively on the fact that they earned a meager stipend whilst they needed to cover their transport to and from their allocated area of work and that they worked a normal workday of 8 hours duration [4] and asserted to the review of the remuneration package to be aligned with labor law in the country.

11.5 Management challenges

The CHWs mentioned that managers are not supporting them in terms of training, shortage of resources, and engaging with the department to transfer their posts to permanent employees.

11.5.1 Inconsistent training

Training of CHWs is not the same; some CHWs have done 10-day courses, and others 59- or 69-day courses, which included HIV counseling and irregular one-off training sessions without opportunities to refresh knowledge which has been reported to demotivate and reduce CHW performance in other LMICs [50]. CHWs refused to conduct certain tasks when they had not been invited to be trained because the training was given to those who were favored and was attached to financial gain [33].

11.5.2 Lack of managerial support and recognition

It was perceived that the challenges of being contract workers and not having enough resources are ongoing. There is an indication that managers are not supporting in terms of the shortage of resources and engaging with the department to transfer their posts to permanent employees. Managers questioned CHW's role perceived by the community as professionals, because of limited training. The managers wanted a planned strategy for CHWs, including career progression and professional regulation, and were concerned about security risk, space, and logistical support. The managers think that CHWs need to be selected based on some criteria, such as education more than matriculation [29].

12. Conclusion

The chapter focused on the definitions of home visits, community health workers and primary health care, overview, the purpose of home visits, historical perspective, advantages and disadvantages, the process of home visits, the challenges perceived by CHWs regarding home visits in the Tshwane district, which were that of community, logistical, occupational, human resource, and managerial.

Acknowledgements

I want to thank the community health workers in the Tshwane District, SG Lourens Nursing College management, supervisors Prof MM Moagi and Prof MD Peu for their guidance and support, and the Department of Health Region C, supervisors of Community Health Workers, Outreach Team Leaders, and Facility managers of the sub-district clinics.

Conflict of interest

The author declares no conflict of interest.

Additional information

Parts of this book chapter are taken from the dissertation titled "Challenges Community Health Workers Perceived Regarding Home Visits in the Tshwane District," authored by Hilda Kawaya, which is available on the University of Pretoria repository platform, dated December 2020. The dissertation has not been peer-reviewed and has not been published.

Author details

Hilda Kawaya
University of Pretoria, Gauteng College of Nursing (GCON) SG Lourens Campus, Pretoria, South Africa

*Address all correspondence to: u18371028@up.ac.za; hkawaya@gmail.com; hilda.kawaya@gcon.ac.za

References

[1] Norful A, Martsolf G, de Jacq K, Poghosyan L. Utilization of registered nurses in primary care teams: A systematic review. International Journal of Nursing Studies. 2017;**74**:15-23

[2] Paintain LS, Willey B, Kedenge S, Sharkey A, Kim J, Buj V, et al. Community health workers and stand-alone or integrated case management of malaria: A systematic literature review. The American Journal of Tropical Medicine and Hygiene. 2014;**91**(3):461-470. DOI: 10.4269/ajtmh.14-0094

[3] Mottiar S, Lodge T. The role of community health workers in supporting South Africa's HIV/AIDS treatment program. African Journal of AIDS Research. 2017;**17**:1. DOI: 10.2989/16085906.1402793

[4] White MS, Govender P, Lister HE. Community health workers lensed through a South African backdrop of two peri-urban communities in KwaZulu-Natal. African Journal of Disability. 2017;**6**:a294. DOI: 10.4102/ajod. v6i0.29

[5] Lerutla M. Gauteng Department of Health, DHS quarterly performance review health workers, recipients' experiences, and constraints to care in South Africa—A pathway to trust. AIDS Care. 2014;**28**(sup4):61-71. DOI: 10.1080/09540121.2016.1195484

[6] Dennill K, Rendall-Mkosi K, King L. Primary Health Care in South Africa. 3rd ed. Cape Town: Oxford University Press; 2013. DOI: 10.1371/journal.pone.0105934

[7] Finello KM, Terteryan A, Riewerts RJ. Home visiting programs: What the primary care clinician should know. Current Problems in Paediatric and Adolescent Health Care. 2016;**46**(4):101-125

[8] Rotheram-Borus MJ, Tomlinson M, Le Roux IM, Harwood JM, Comulada S, et al. A cluster randomised controlled effectiveness trial evaluating perinatal home visiting among south African mothers/infants. PLoS One. 2014;**9**(10):e105934

[9] Ichikawa K, Fujiwara T, Nakayama T. Correction: Effectiveness of home visits in pregnancy as a public health measure to improve birth outcomes. PLoS One. 2016;**11**(3):e0152354. DOI: 10.1371/journal.pone.0152354

[10] Mayo-Wilson E, Grant S, Burton J, Parsons A, Underhill K, et al. Preventive home visits for mortality, morbidity, and institutionalization in older adults: A systematic review and meta-analysis. PLoS One. 2014;**9**(3):e89257. DOI: 10.1371/journal.pone.0089257

[11] Mascarenas DN, Wurzburger R, Garcia BN, Tomedi A, Mwanthi MA. The promise of home visitation by community health workers in rural Kenya: A protective effect that reduces neonatal illness. Education for Health. 2015, 2015;**28**(3):181-186

[12] Seutloali T, Napoles L, Bam N. Community health workers in Lesotho: Experiences of health promotion activities. African Journal of Primary Health Care & Family Medicine. 2018, 2018;**10**(1):8, ISSN 2071-2936

[13] You H, Chen J, Bogg L, Wu Y, Duan S, Ye C, et al. PLOS xl. study on the factors associated with postpartum visits in rural China. PLOS ONE. 2013;**8**(2):e55955. DOI: 10.1371/journal.pone.0055955

[14] Bheekie A, Bradley H. Re-engineering of South Africa's primary health care system: Where is the pharmacist? South African Family

Practice. 2016;**58**(6):242-248. DOI: 10.1080/20786190.2016.1186365

[15] Rabkin M, Mutiti A, Mwansa J, Macheka T, Austin-Evelyn K, El-Sadr WM. 2015. Re-engineering Primary Health Care: A Formative Process Evaluation of rPHC implementation in King Sabata Dalundyebo sub-district in the Eastern Cape Province of South Africa. Available from: http:// academiccommons.

[16] Pillay Y, Barron P. 2011.The Implementation of PHC Re-engineering in South Africa. Public Health Association of South Africa. Available from: http://www.phasa.org.za/the-implementation-of-phc-reengineering-in-South-Africa/

[17] Grant M, Wilford A, Haskins L, Phakathi S, Mntambo N, Horwood CM. Trust of community health workers influences the acceptance of community-based maternal and child health services. African Journal of Primary Health Care & Family Medicine. 2017, 2017;**9**(1):1281

[18] Backes DS, Haeffner L, Dorin L, et al. Meaning of home visits to Brazilian health students. Nurse Care. Open Access Journal. 2017, 2017;**4**(1):358-363. DOI: 10.15406/ncoaj

[19] Shaban IA, Al-Awamreh K, Mohammad K, Gharaibeh H. Postnatal women's perspectives on the feasibility of introducing postpartum home visits: A Jordanian study. Home Health Care Services Quarterly. 2018;**37**:3. DOI: 10.1080/01621424.2018.1454865

[20] WHO. The World Health Report 2014. Primary Health Care - Now More than Ever. Vol. 26. Geneva: World Health Organization; 2014. Available from: http://www.who.int/whr/2014/whr14_en.pdf

[21] Novins D, Meyer A, Beltangady M. Contextual issues for implementation and evaluation of home-visitation programs for American Indian and Alaska native communities: An introduction to the tribal maternal, infant, and early childhood home visiting program. Infant Mental Health Journal. 2018;**39, 2018**(3):259-264. DOI: 10.1002/imhj.21705

[22] Sitrin D, Guenther T, Waiswa P, Namutamba S, Namazzi G, Sharma S, et al. Improving newborn care practices through home visits: Lessons from Malawi, Nepal, Bangladesh, and Uganda. Global Health Action. 2015;**8**:1. DOI: 10.3402/gha. v8.23963

[23] Salami KK, Brieger WR. Service delivery and coverage in primary healthcare in a community-based project in Ibadan, Nigeria. African Journal of Primary Health & Family Medicine. 2014;**6**(1):545

[24] Magin P, Catzikiris N, Tapley A, Morgan S, Holliday EG, Ball J, et al. Home visits and nursing home visits by earlier career GPs: A cross-sectional study. Family Practice. 2017;**1**:77-82. DOI: 10.1093/fampra/cmw099

[25] Voigt K, Bojanowski K, Taché S, Voigt R, Bergmann A. Home visits in Primary care: Contents and organization in daily practice. Study protocol of a cross-sectional study. BMJ Open. 2016;**6**(2):e008209. DOI: 10.1136/BMJ open-2015-008209

[26] Liimatta H, Lampela P, Laitinen-Parkkonen P, Pitkala KH. Effects of preventative home visits on older people's use and costs of health care services: A systematic review'. European Geriatric Medicine. 2016;**7**(6):571-580. DOI: 10.1016/j.eurger.2016.08.006

[27] Darikwa P. An exploration of the perceptions of Community Health

Workers on the enablers and barriers to providing services in Nyanga District, Zimbabwe [master thesis]. University of Witwatersrand; 2016

[28] Wells S, O'Neill M, Rogers J, Blaine K, Hoffman A, McBride S, et al. Nursing-led home visits posthospitalization for children with medical complexity. Journal of Pediatric Nursing. 2017;**34**:10-16

[29] Moosa S, Derese A, Peersman W. Insights of health district managers on the implementation of primary health care outreach teams in Johannesburg, South Africa: A descriptive study with focus group discussions. Human Resources for Health. 2017;**15**(1):7

[30] Perry HB, Zulliger R, Rogers MM. Community health workers in low-, middle-, and high-income countries: An overview of their history, recent evolution, and current effectiveness. Annual Review of Public Health. 2014;**35**:399-421. DOI: 10.1146/annurev-publhealth-032013-182354

[31] Kane S, Kok M, Ormel H, Otiso L, Sidat M, Namakhoma I, et al. Limits and opportunities to community health worker empowerment: A multi-country comparative study. Social Science & Medicine. 2016;**164**:27-34. DOI: 10.1016/j.socscimed.2016.07.019. Epub, PMID: 27459022

[32] Mhlongo EM, Lutge E. The roles, responsibilities, and perceptions of community health workers and ward-based primary health care outreach teams (WBPHCOTs) in South Africa: A scoping review protocol. Systematic Reviews. 2019;**8**(1):1-7. DOI: 10.1186/s13643-019-1114-5

[33] Kok MC, Dieleman M, Taegtmeyer M, Broerse JEW, Kane SS, Ormel H, et al. Which intervention design factors influence the performance of community health workers in low- and middle-income countries? A systematic review. Health Policy Plan. 2015;**30**(9):1207-1227

[34] Zulliger R, Moshabela M, Schneider H. "She is my teacher and if it was not for her, I would be dead": Exploration of rural south African community health workers' information, education, and communication activities. AIDS Care. 2014;**26**(5):626-632

[35] LeRoux K, LeRoux I, Mbewu N, Davis E. The role of community health workers in the re-engineering of primary health care in rural Eastern Cape. South African Family Practice. 2015;**57**:2. DOI: 10.1080/20786190.2014.977063

[36] Kelly JD, Frankfurter R, Lurton G, et al. Evaluation of a community-based ART programme after tapering home visits in rural Sierra Leone: A 24-month retrospective study. SAHARA-J: Journal of Social Aspects of HIV/AIDS. 2018;**15**(1):138-145. DOI: 10.1080/17290376.2018.1527244

[37] Nkosi-Gondwe T, Robberstad B, Blomberg B, Phiri KS, Lange S. Introducing post-discharge malaria chemoprevention (PMC) for management of severe anemia in Malawian children: A qualitative study of community health workers' perceptions and motivation. BMC Health Services Research. 2018;**18**:1-5. DOI: 10.1186/S12913-018-3791-5

[38] Pillay Y. PHC Engineering in South Africa: Are we making progress? Public Health Association of South Africa. Newsletter. 29 February 2012. Available from: http://www.phasa.org.za/articles/phc-re-engineering-in-south-africa-are-we-making-progress.html

[39] World Health Organization. Declaration of the First Global

Ministerial Conference on Healthy Lifestyles and Noncommunicable Disease Control. Moscow: World Health Organization; 2013

[40] Lawn JE, Bhutta ZA, Wall SN, Peterson S, Daviaud E. Cadres, content, and costs for community-based care for mothers and newborns from seven countries: Implications for universal health coverage. Health Policy, and Planning. 2017;**32**(suppl_1):i1-i5. DOI: 10.1093/heapol/czx104

[41] Agarwal S, Anaba U, Abuya T, Kintu R, Casseus A, Hossain S, et al. Understanding incentive preferences of community health workers using discrete choice experiments: Multi-country protocol for Kenya, Uganda, Bangladesh, and Haiti. BMJ Open. 2019, 2019;**9**:e033601. DOI: 101136/bmjopen-2019-033601

[42] Fusheini A, Eyles J. Achieving universal health coverage in South Africa through a district health system approach: Conflicting ideologies of health care provision. BMC Health Services Research. 2016;**16**:558. DOI: 10.1186/s12913-016-1797-4

[43] De Neve J-W, Garrison-Desany H, Andrews KG, Sharara N, Boudreaux C, Gill R, et al. Harmonization of community health worker programs for HIV: A four-country qualitative study in Southern Africa. PLoS Medicine. 2017;**14**(8):e1002374. DOI: 10.1371/journal.pmed.1002374

[44] Ayiasi R, Kolsteren P, Batwala V, Criel B, Orach CG. Effect of village health team home visits and Mobile phone consultations on maternal and Newborn care practices in Masindi and Kiryandongo, Uganda: A community-intervention trial. PLoS One. 2016;**11**(4):e0153051. DOI: 10.1371/journal.pone.0153051

[45] Diomande MN. The perceived role of Community Health Workers in Voluntary Medical Male Circumcision demands creation [master thesis]. Johannesburg: University of Witwatersrand; 2019

[46] Busza J, Dauya E, Bandason T, Simms V, Chikwari CD, Makamba M, et al. The role of community health workers in improving HIV treatment outcomes in children: Lessons learned from the ZENITH trial in Zimbabwe. Health Policy and Planning. 2018;**33**(3):328-334. DOI: 10.1093/heapol/czx187

[47] Josephson K, Guerrero G, Coddington C. Supporting the Early Childhood Workforce at Scale: The Cuna Más Home Visiting Program in Peru. Washington, D.C: Juta & Company Ltd; 2017

[48] Clark MJ. Population and Community Health Nursing. 6th ed. Hoboken, New Jersey: Pearson Education; 2015

[49] Ndaba T, Taylor M, Mabaso M. Training and evaluation of community health workers (CHWs): Towards improving maternal and newborn survival in an urban setting in KwaZulu-Natal, South Africa. The Open Public Health Journal. 2019;**12**:406-413

[50] Ozano K, Simkhada P, Thann K, et al. Improving local health through community health workers in Cambodia: Challenges and solutions. Human Resource for Health. 2018;**16**:2. DOI: 10.1186/s12960-017-0262-8

Section 4

Artificial Intelligence and Telemedicine in Health Care

Chapter 10

Reinforcing Positive Cognitive States with Machine Learning: An Experimental Modeling for Preventive Healthcare

Swapnil Morande, Veena Tewari and Kanwal Gul

Abstract

Societal evolution has resulted in a complex lifestyle where we give most attention to our physical health leaving psychological health less prioritized. Considering the complex relationship between stress and psychological well-being, this study bases itself on the cognitive states experienced by us. The presented research offers insight into how state-of-the-art technologies can be used to support positive cognitive states. It makes use of the brain-computer interface (BCI) that drives the data collection using electroencephalography (EEG). The study leverages data science to devise machine learning (ML) model to predict the corresponding stress levels of an individual. A feedback loop using "Self Quantification" and "Nudging" offer real-time insights about an individual. Such a mechanism can also support the psychological conditioning of an individual where it does not only offer spatial flexibility and cognitive assistance but also results in enhanced self-efficacy. Being part of quantified self-movement, such an experimental approach could showcase personalized indicators to reflect a positive cognitive state. Although ML modeling in such a data-driven approach might experience reduced diagnostic sensitivity and suffer from observer variability, it can complement psychosomatic treatments for preventive healthcare.

Keywords: BCI, EEG, machine learning, well-being, positive cognitive state

1. Introduction

What if, one day, you wear a hat that would read the negative emotions and alters your thoughts by enacting small tweaks so that you could experience joy? It sounds like a script for a sci-fi movie, but it could also be the future of the healthcare industry. Stress, anxiety, and depression are major global issues; however, less importance is being paid due to their psychosomatic nature. Depression is a disease of modernity—major depressive disorder (MDD), stress, attention deficit hyperactivity disorder (ADHD); our lifestyle, industrial revolution 4.0, work-life imbalance, social media, gadgets, and eating disorders are potential reasons behind deteriorating psychological health [1–3]. Psychological health refers to how we behave, feel, and think.

Furthermore, it determines how skillfully we can manage stressors that are part of our lives. Poor psychological well-being will not only affect our personal life but also have a hazardous effect on our work-life as well [4].

Our cognitive state of mind is continuously affected by experiences at the workplace and by the choices, we make in our personal lives. According to the WHO, 280 million people around the world are suffering from depression [5]. Depression is challenging our everyday life in many ways: unproductivity at work, poor relationship management, loss of interest in life, and at its worst, it can even marshal a person to suicide. The common knowledge is that depression and stress are the same things while both concepts are different. Stress—caused by stressors, i.e., negative cognitive state or emotion/feelings—can be beneficial at times [6]. On the other hand, depression is a ramification of chronic stress, which causes mood disorder, existential crises, and disinterest in everyday tasks and makes us feel sad. Due to the evolution of society, stressors have arisen because of a complex lifestyle. In the process of fulfilling our wish list, our psychological health suffers, causing enormous side effects. Our physical health remains important, but psychological health takes a back seat. Psychological health deteriorates because of chronic stress, which is undoubtedly the genesis of depression and negative cognitive states.

Stress is a complex feeling and stressors are convoluted. The traditional way of understating the potentiality of stressors is a change in lifestyle, medication, and/or talk/cognitive behavioral therapy (CBT); such activities require time, money, effort, and accessibility. These therapies can be used to treat depression, but the techniques and tenure of each therapy are different from the another [7]. This raises the question of the long-term efficacy of these therapies. Apart from long-term efficacy, another problem arises that one must have resources and time to get these therapies. Most of them are offered in 1:1 sessions. It should also be considered that in developed countries there are certain protocols developed for the availability of therapists, convenience for taking sessions, and awareness campaigns to eradicate taboos from society about mental health and mental illness, while in developing countries the case is the opposite [8, 9]. Nevertheless, these protocols cannot reach the masses.

Apart from talk therapies, medications and meditations are also used to cure depression and stress.

A systematic review of meditation therapy on 1173 patients having acute and subacute depressive symptoms concluded that meditation may have positive effects on the patients while heterogeneity of techniques and trial designs limits the treatment's generalizability [10]. On the other hand, medications/drugs are a short-term solution to ease stress, and it contains major side effects. If the goal is to promote well-being rather than simply treat sickness, mental health providers must apply novel techniques to assessment and therapy [11].

Patients have typically been treated by medical personnel as passive recipients of their treatment in the healthcare industry [12]. It is necessary to reevaluate this passive viewpoint, which has been pervasive in the healthcare industry [13]. Additionally, research based on well-being needs to be integrated and applied so that health practitioners may involve their patients and provide better results. One of the most debated topics in today's healthcare scenario is how to employ technology to improve access to and quality of care, as well as the patient experience [14]. Technologies such as A.I. and Healthcare IoT have been widely deployed in a variety of industries, with healthcare being one of them. As technology can play its role by offering affordable and accessible solutions. It does not limit itself to physical health [15] and can go beyond to serve as a critical element for reinforcing positive cognitive states.

Today, technology is capable to change the dynamics of the traditional way of dealing with depression, anxiety, and stress. Following these advances in technology allows us to study and analyze the brain more accurately than before. One of the breakthroughs is electroencephalography (EEG) was commonly used to detect a tumor, epilepsy, sleep disorder, brain death, and coma. Brain-computer interface (BCI) is a system that connects a human mind to a computer to link the brain/brain activity to a computer. BCI is a noninvasive system that has used brain signals to offer a communication system. Apart from improving the sensorimotor function of humans, BCI also offers therapeutic paradigms. The elements of BCI are the detection of brain activity, categorizing it, give feedback in real-time [16].

BCIs are not limited to the recording paradigms but also consider the "will" of the user who generates signals. The "will" of a user is divided into three categories: 1) the subject is willingly producing a signal for which the spontaneous BCI system would be used, 2) the subject is being exposed to certain stimuli produced by the evoked BCI system and generates a signal, and 3) the subject uses normal arousal activity or signal produced by a brain of the subject for which passive BCI system would be used. Building on studies of value co-creation and smart technologies, scientists are considering the opportunities that how smart technologies and tech-enabled healthcare can help practitioners and patients. As proposed in this chapter brain-computer interface can enable patients to track themselves and can be used to read the data provided by the patient. A.I. leverages digitized data to provide smart nudges to prevent behavioral risk factors. Catapulted by the stream of data, the A.I. interacts with people based on their lifestyle and emotional states and permits expression of autonomy for reinforcing positive cognitive states, which increases their self-efficacy for preventive healthcare.

2. Literature review

2.1 Psychosomatic health

We live in volatile times with constant stress, where the source of stress are personal relationships, workplace pressure, and financial problems, together known as "stressors" [6]. We frequently hold onto this stress, allowing its negative effects to build up. Such circumstances may result in serious health issues such as anxiety and depression [17]. When compared to the number of individuals who experience it, research on mental health is inadequate, and this disparity is especially glaring for low- and middle-income nations [18]. Psychosomatic health reflects both mind and body. At any given time, our mental health influences our physical health. Certain physical conditions and diseases are especially vulnerable to being exacerbated by emotional variables like stress and worry. Considering this, it is crucial to pay attention to both physical as well as mental health. The balance of both can result in the well-being of an individual's health. The link between physical and psychological health is significant and the prevalence of mental diseases is rising [19]. It has grown to be a serious public health problem that affects people worldwide.

Mental health professionals must use cutting-edge techniques for assessment and counseling if the intention is to promote well-being rather than only treat illness [11]. Research into mental illness is developing quickly, with help from studies in the fields of genetics, genomics, psychiatry, and epidemiology, among others. Clinical practice should continue to be informed by these advancements at an exponential rate. Patients have typically been treated by medical personnel as passive recipients of their treatment in the healthcare industry [12]. The challenge is also to apply and integrate the body of research on well-being so that health practitioners may involve their patients and achieve better outcomes.

2.2 Constructs of well-being

Well-being is a multifaceted construct that is affected by human sentiments of feeling happy, cheerful, and excited [20]. Research states that psychological well-being has cognitive appraisals [21] and can be operationalized with indicators that represent positively balanced emotion as indicated in **Figure 1**.

Stress levels have a deleterious impact on psychological health [22] and there exists strong evidence to support the relationship between stress and psychological health [23]. Data have also shown a considerable negative correlation between psychological well-being and perceived job stress. Among the psychosocial risk factors frequently examined concerning poor health are anger, anxiety, depression, and social isolation. A positive cognitive state is concerned with positive psychological states (e.g., happiness), and positive psychological traits (e.g., interests). Concern for positive health leads to an examination of health assets, and individual-level factors that represent positive cognitive states [24–26].

2.3 Significance of technology

Replication and the use of technology to enhance the patient experience, access to treatment, and care quality are one of the most contested issues in today's healthcare environment [14]. Technologies such as IoT have been widely applied across industries including healthcare [27]. Its capabilities are expected to expedite medical procedures, provide individuals with more control over their medical information, and improve the general quality of medical results [28].

Early healthcare research was limited to clinicians, psychologists, behavioral scientists, and therapists, but today, mapping of brain activity is possible through computers; initiated with functional magnetic resonance imagining (fMRI), a radiation-less, noninvasive, and accessible technological breakthrough. A recent innovation in brain imagining includes transcranial magnetic (TCM) stimulation

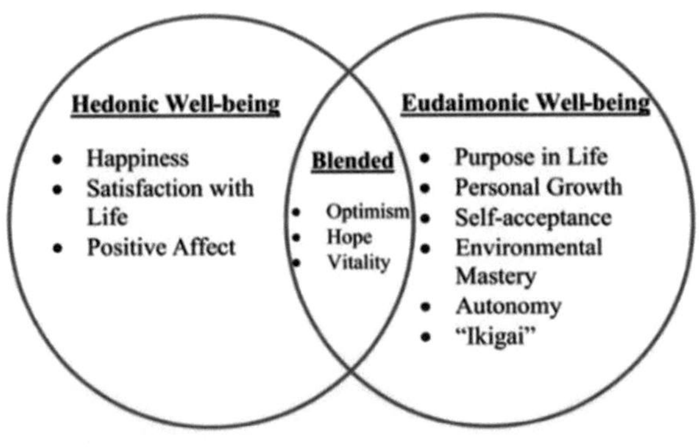

Figure 1.
Conception and categorization of psychological well-being.

a coil placed on the head of the subject that generates a magnetic field and stimulus that allows the subject to perform some activity through the mind without using peripheral nerves and muscles. At the same time, today, EEG-based brain-computer interphase (BCI) is also being used to study brain activity. Initially, the technology was used to allow people—physically disabled—to perform their routine tasks using brain signals connected with BCI that controls robotic limbs. As a matter of course, scientists also worked on the assumption that "if a human can control the machine through its brain, then it is also possible to control the brain through a machine" [29].

BCI can record brain signals in two ways: 1) noninvasive recording of brain signals through the scalp using electroencephalography (EEG), functional magnetic resonance imaging (fMRI), and near-infrared spectroscopy (NIRS); 2) invasive recording using electrocorticography (ECoG) by placing electrodes on the surface of the cortex and microelectrode arrays placing within the cortex or inserted into a single cell.

The above approaches have their merits and demerits. Invasive technologies are associated with more risk due to the requirement of the surgical method, but it gives a higher signal-to-noise ratio. On the contrary, noninvasive technologies are more popular than nonsurgical methods for their cost-efficiency, portability, and safety purposes, however, the quality of the signal-to-noise ratio—the intensity of brain signals to noise intensity—is lower as compared to invasive technology. Thus, exploring the opportunities and challenges of artificial intelligence (AI) in healthcare it can be confirmed that A.I. can be used to perform diagnostics and assisted well-being [30]. It indicates how technology can relinquish ubiquitous connectivity for the betterment of health services [31].

Technology is the driving force behind the healthcare industry, and it dramatically predicts the future. While we might speculate about healthcare trends in the future, we must take proactive measures to guarantee the best results for society [32]. Although implementing cutting-edge medical technology can be expensive, research indicates that the social value of living longer and healthier lives should be prioritized over the expense [33].

A.I. facilitates value creation by enhancing the resource exchange process resulting in expanded interaction capabilities and co-created value for both parties. With the potential for value co-creation, A.I. enables service providers to attain an unprecedented level of reliability [34]. The focus shifts from individual technologies (and devices) to the socio-material practices enabled by the application of the A.I. and IoM in healthcare [35]. A.I. approaches will mature and could help mental health practitioners redefine mental issues more objectively and personalize therapies [36]. More effort is required to bridge the divide between mental health clinical care and AI research. Implementing artificial intelligence in healthcare is a compelling concept that has the potential to lead to major advances in accomplishing real-time and tailored treatment at lower costs [37]. Even though these systems face numerous methodological and ethical issues, they have the potential to permit large-scale data collecting far beyond the scope of typical research laboratory settings [38]. From deep learning to control of health management systems, its informatics-driven techniques and active physician guidance in treatment decisions cannot be ignored [39]. A system is a complex object made up of interdependent parts that interact with one another and with their environments and it exhibits continuous evolution by assimilating new attributes for emergence [40]. Systems theory can be applied in service science to investigate phenomena from a holistic approach [41] where observed reality can be perceived as an integrated and interacting unicum of phenomena [42].

Connections between cognitive technologies and humans can establish intricate service networks with novel value propositions [43].

2.4 Quantified self

Self-tracking, commonly referred to as "quantified self," is increasingly popular in the healthcare industry [44]. Several people are embracing self-quantification where they can receive "self-knowledge via numbers" in the hope of improving their well-being [45]. Self-tracking technology has raised expectations, if not outright hype, for helping people manage their health risks and promote optimal wellness [46]. However, because of the discrepancies between personal experiences and self-tracking data, strong expectations could not always be realized. This is a concern if people are expected to participate more in the collection and analysis of their personal data for their health and well-being. The ability to self-track would translate into the management of patient health and ease the process of making wise therapeutic decisions [47]. One of the main characteristics of self-tracking is how users respond to self-tracking data. The findings show that mentality plays a crucial role in defining the self-tracking experience. Even though self-tracking positively affects customers' impressions of personalization [48], its data-driven and quantifiable features might occasionally result in excessive self-monitoring. This could put more pressure on the user to perform following strict health standards, which could cause feelings of inadequacy and make it difficult for them to enjoy exercising [49]. Meanwhile, several studies have noted an increase in self-efficacy in relation to self-quantification [50, 51].

2.5 Nudge theory

"Nudge theory" proposed that an intervention aimed at modifying the cognitive boundaries may gradually alter the actions of an individual [52]. When nudge seems to be people's declared self-interests, such intervention need not deal with the negativity of traditional enforcement. The behavioral sciences have created nudge to change behavior, which challenges the conventional use of regulation in public health policy to address modifiable individual-level behaviors. Nudging interventions are marked as "a rearrangement of a decision context that softly encourages a specific choice" [53] as well as "physical modifications in the choice architecture that predictably influence people's choices." These interventions change how humans make choices, which contributes to cognitive biases—that is, changing how options are presented to individuals—so that people's cognitive biases drive them to act in their own best interests, the best interests of societies, or both. While decision-making biases can be used to encourage individual health behavior, straightforward interventions can encourage people to make the best possible decisions for their health without affecting the decision-makers' freedom of choice [54].

Further, nudging techniques have been applied for improving user engagement in mental health and reinforcing positive cognitive states using technologies [55]. In the assessment of the self-tracking process, in many use cases, the individual benefits through a sustained engagement in the process and use of self-tracking technologies [56]. According to this study, routine tracking may enhance patients' self-efficacy and help them develop their self-management skills more effectively than event-driven recording. Both self-efficacy and self-management skills are linked to better health outcomes [57].

2.6 Positive cognitive states

Reinforcing positive cognitive states is synonymous with a condition of flourishing that includes health, happiness, and prosperity and includes an individual's emotions as well as their overall assessment of life satisfaction. It is a key result in health research that assists in determining the effectiveness of therapies and treatments as well as understanding patients' experiences [58]. A review of literature by Ref. [59] suggests positive cognitive states through well-being encompass diverse experiences that include positive affective states, low levels of negative affective states as well as good psychosomatic health. The definition of well-being should include a positive psychological state rather than only the absence of mental illness [60]. Individuals' well-being—as healthcare customers' perceptions—is a highly desired outcome of interest to both researchers and practitioners [61]. This study examines positive cognitive states which include a person's feelings like despair and anxiety, from the perspective of preventive healthcare. The latest pandemic's psychological effects necessitate the creation of an intervention to enhance mental health [62, 63]. The positive feelings that are impacted by stressors [64] from the outside world could be used to gauge one's level of well-being [3]. When subjected to stressors, the "stress" underlines the response by the heart that outweighs the individual's perceived ability to cope with it [59, 65]. Despite being a subjective notion, well-being does reflect the effects of stress, and [66] confirmed that a decrease in stress results in improved well-being. As a result, a person's well-being can be determined by how they react to changing pressures and retain positive cognitive states [67]. It should be a top priority to look at the aspect of preventive healthcare and to do this, it is crucial to track each person's degree of stress [68].

2.7 Research gap and objective

Based on the review of the literature, we understand that the gap exists in finding the role and impact of the technology on reinforcing positive cognitive states. Hence the research objective for the given study is to ascertain whether positive emotions contribute to well-being and check how that translates into organizational productivity.

3. Research method

The presented research is based on an exploratory study that is fueled by qualitative data collection and its A.I.-driven analysis. Its "Mixed mode" approach has been well-established for merging complex research designs [69]. In this study, it was important to understand whether psychological health affects physical health. Upon confirmation, it needed to establish whether the involvement of technology can enhance well-being. Finally, the last stage looked at emotional states and energy levels on workplace productivity. Hence the research methodology adopted "Sequential Multiple Methodology" that had been divided into four stages [70]. These stages were utilized to observe the occurrence of a phenomenon to improve psychological well-being. A statistical analysis tool was utilized for the multivariate analysis required to fulfill the research objective.

The machine learning (ML) modeling supported developing illustrations of essential trends and variations presented in the given study. It operated on the data retrieved using electroencephalography (EEG). A device that made it possible is called a brain-computer interface [71]. With five EEG electrodes at the AF3, AF4, T7, Pz, and two reference electrodes, BCI recorded brainwaves and produced precise band activity with defined frequencies. Alpha waves are a representation of the brain's natural "relaxed" and "alert" states. A beta wave is connected to active attention and thinking activities. Drowsiness, arousal, and meditation are all characteristics of theta activity. Gamma rhythms develop when distinct groups of neurons work together to carry out challenging cognitive or physical tasks. It reflected upon the emotional states experienced by the subjects. Considering the complex nature and interactions of brain signals A.I. played a significant role in this stage. As EEG data have thousands of instances recorded in a second; it becomes extremely difficult for health professionals to reflect on the tremendous volume of generated data.

Simultaneously, quantitative data metrics were collected from the subjects in the form of a questionnaire that included both quantitative and qualitative questions. Both BCI data and survey data were used to understand workplace productivity. The construct for depicting "Workplace Productivity" included stress (represented by age, lifestyle, and emotional states) and energy levels (using sleep pattern and circadian rhythm). Given study deployed "stratified sampling" that has put a narrow focus on similar characteristics of the research population that was collected from India in consideration of ethical guidelines. Power analysis for linear regression was completed in G*Power using an alpha of 0.05, a power of 0.80, a large effect size ($p = .5$), and two tails to establish an adequate sample size. Based on the aforementioned assumptions, the ideal sample size is 26 [72].

3.1 Data modeling

The latter part of the study was used for ML modeling using a decision tree as a statistical technique. Considering a large number of data points and to derive real-time insights, the presented research opted for data science-driven techniques using ML-driven modeling [73].

Although such data modeling provides greater depth of the impact of predictors on the dependent variable psychosomatic construct can be complex to evaluate. This is because the brain generates relevant waves multiple times in an instant. It could even go as far as thousands of instances per second. Hence for a particular instance, the value of stress keeps on changing with interest, relaxation, excitement, focus, and engagement as mediators. Thus, evaluating the state of health of an individual as a particular instance calls for a holistic approach in consideration of the signal emitted by other cortices of the human brain. Such calculations could get very complex; hence

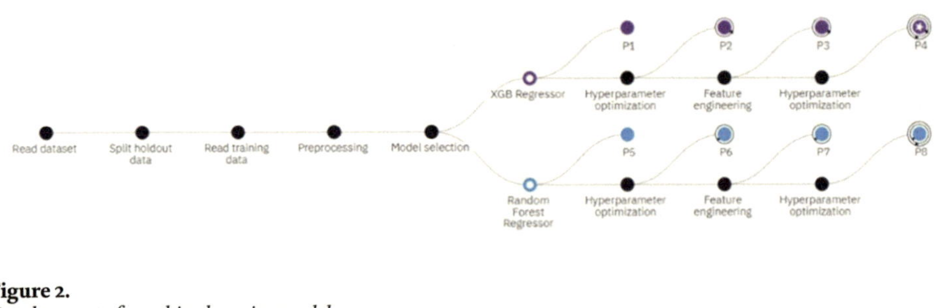

Figure 2.
Development of machine learning model.

in the given study, machine learning is used to predict the possible instance based on the historical data and patterns.

As shown in **Figure 2,** the power of prediction granted by data science can make an individual proactive toward their state of health, and the same has been used in the study as a preventive and personalized way to attain positive cognitive states [37].

4. Findings

The "Sequential Multiple Methodology" in this research aligns four stages of the study including the pilot study that draws insights using both qualitative and quantitative techniques. A pilot study shows that mental health has a certain impact on the individual physical health **(Stage I),** confirming the existence of the "Psychosomatic" nature of the health aspect. The variables in play include—Psychological_Issue, Subconscious_Mind, Bio_Signatures, Physical_Issue, Conscious_Mind, Therapeutic_Intervention, Role_of_Technology, Personality_Dimensions, and Psychosomatic_Health. The same can be proven through "Pearson Correlation" that displays a significant positive correlation was observed between Psychological_Issue and Physical_Issue.

The next stage **(Stage II)** cascades the above finding to identify the role of technology on individuals' well-being. Using qualitative illustrations such as "Sentiment Analysis" and "Co-occurrence Table." Both these techniques make sure that case study selection stays balanced and with minimal bias. It identifies eHealth as an emerging trend and supports the application of A.I. for the exploration of cognitive states. The same was confirmed with qualitative comments from the health professionals and relevant case studies were analyzed using qualitative content analysis (QCA). **Stage III** of the research design—being the most critical one—treats Psychological Well-being as a multidimensional construct, and as a product of emotions, happiness, and positive affect. During this stage, the results of the linear regression model were significant, $F(12,1509) = 1584.37$, $p < .001$, $R2 = 0.93$, indicating that approximately 93% of the variance in STRESS is explainable with the Regression Equation. It verifies the fact that sustained stress and negative feelings experienced by a person can potentially affect individuals' well-being.

In this part of the study, a data-driven machine learning model (Refer to **Figure 3**) was used to bridge the information silos and create a personalized model to assist with stress management. It reflects that, with the self-learning technology offering insights in real-time, it would be easier to maintain or improve psychological well-being. Furthermore, this stage also confirms that positive emotions contribute to well-being. In such an exploration, we can gain a greater understanding of how technology contributes to the improvement of well-being.

Workplace productivity is explored in **Stage IV** of the research design, where, as an emotional state, "Focus" plays an important role. It uses Spearman correlation among variables including AGE, BMI, FOCUS, CIRCADIAN_RHYTHM, GENDER, STATE_OF_HEALTH, STRESS, ENERGY_LEVEL, LIFESTYLE, ENGAGEMENT, SLEEP, and OBSERVED_PRODUCTIVITY. A significant negative correlation was observed between FOCUS and OBSERVED_PRODUCTIVITY ($r = -0.12$, $p < .001$, 95% CI = [−0.17, −0.07]).

The correlation coefficient between FOCUS and OBSERVED_PRODUCTIVITY was—0.12, indicating a small effect size. This correlation indicates that as FOCUS increases, OBSERVED_PRODUCTIVITY tends to decrease.

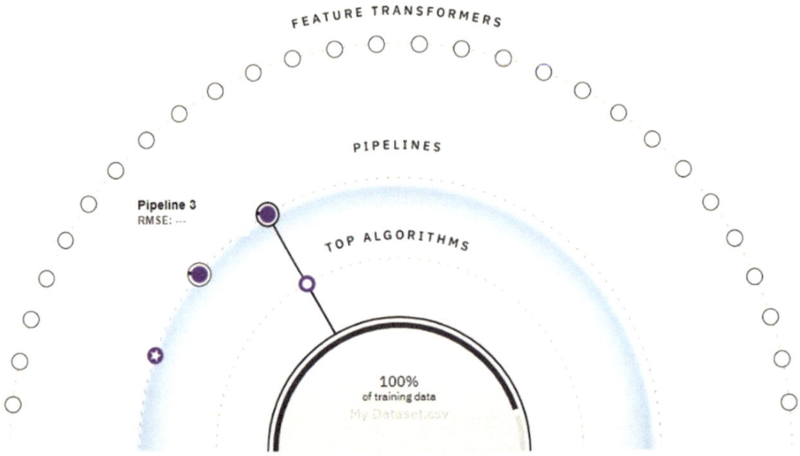

Figure 3.
Feature transformation of ML model.

Using establish constructs the energy levels of a person can be understood using the historical data on circadian rhythm and sleep patterns. Optimal stress and energy levels were used to measure workplace productivity [74]. In this process, stress is moderated by engagement, interest, focus, and relaxation states. Self-quantification (of cognitive indicators) can be augmented using A.I. where nudges dynamically become smart nudges that offer positive cognitive states. Additionally, this stage reviews prior academic literature to reflect on how workplace well-being drives organizational performance. As a result of the literature review conducted for this study, we understand that allows us to reflect on the co-created value for an organization through individual well-being.

Observing the effect of emotional states and psychological well-being.

- From Stage III of the research design, we can observe that stress levels are strongly correlated with the emotional states of individuals.
- There are three variables involved in this process: stress, interest, and relaxation.
- Self-quantification is an effective method for maintaining psychological well-being, which is a product of a person's emotional state.

Observing the impact of psychological well-being and workplace productivity.

- Using Stage IV data, we can determine that an individual's Focus directly impacts their workplace productivity.
- A mediator in this process is "Focus," while moderators include "Body's clock" and "Energy levels."
- Additionally, the current knowledge may be linked to relevant academic literature to conclude that workplace productivity has a direct impact on organizational performance.

5. Discussions

The research addresses the evolution of practices driven by these technologies and how they advance the multiple aspects of healthcare. The capability and scalability of the technological platform are likely to support inclusive and sustainable enhancement in psychosomatic healthcare. In this study, different emotional reactions were evoked from the subjects during data collection. EEG frequencies from five different cerebral cortices were included in the data that was gathered: ALPHA, BETA (H), BETA (L), GAMMA, and THETA frequencies. By identifying the significance of each frequency, scaled values were calculated for attributes such as engagement, focus, excitement, interest, relaxation, and stress. Using data science, a machine learning (ML) model was trained to identify the probable effect of "Stress" as a target value for prediction.

The algorithm learned from the data and predicted the target values with higher accuracy, as shown in **Figure 4**. Thus, findings from the study largely shed light on the occurrence of psychosomatic illness and the potential contribution of technology to improving psychological health. Later, through data-driven research, the study analyses emotional states and personal well-being. For the fulfillment of this study, two constructs were used to identify Stress and predict Productivity. The construct of stress relied on the degree of "Interest" and "Relaxation," while the construct of productivity was dependent on the "Focus" and "Engagement" levels of an individual.

5.1 Cognitive attributes

An electroencephalograph (EEG) reflects neural oscillations generated by the human brain. These brainwaves can be read using a brain-computer interface (BCI) and converted into scaled values for analysis. Such a setup can be used to enhance psychosomatic health using a data-driven model. Measures including age, state of health, engagement, relaxation, interest, and focus significantly affect the stress levels of a person, of which, the relaxation and interest levels are the most prominent ones. In the healthcare ecosystem, brainwaves interact with applied therapeutic Interventions and integrate resources to reflect on current lifestyle and state of health.

Measures	Holdout score	Cross validation score
Root mean squared error	0.029	0.027
R squared	0.929	0.939
Explained variance	0.930	0.939
Mean squared error	0.001	0.001
Mean squared log error	0.000	0.000
Mean absolute error	0.019	0.020
Median absolute error	0.014	0.014
Root mean squared log error	0.020	0.020

Figure 4.
Machine learning model performance.

Feature name	Transformation	Feature importance
INTEREST	None	100.00%
RELAXATION	None	45.00%
INTERVENTION DENSITY	None	6.00%
SLEEP	None	5.00%
NewFeature_1	nxor(ENGAGEMENT,RELAXATION)	5.00%
NewFeature_9	nxor(INTEREST,FOCUS)	4.00%
LIFESTYLE	None	4.00%
AGE	None	3.00%
NewFeature_2	nxor(ENGAGEMENT,INTEREST)	3.00%

Figure 5.
Summary of ML model's features importance.

This provides an individual with a relaxed state of mind releasing stress. With such an approach, therapists can diagnose and offer prognosis of stress levels for the betterment of cognitive states. Using artificial intelligence and managing individual attributes, it is possible to achieve optimal stress levels. The emotional and physiological response to unmanageable and unpredictable circumstances is perceived as "Psychological Stress." It is a reflection of the intense stress caused by difficult cognitive tasks completed under time and social constraints. It is established that factors connected to "Individual Lifestyle," "Brainwaves," and "Therapeutic Intervention" affect an individual's stress levels based on the low p-value (.05) of the indicators. Age, gender, and state of health (Prior) are uncontrollable, as data analysis reveals; however, the intervention density can be changed to induce varying levels of stress in a person. The ML model summary report presented in **Figure 5** confirms that psychologists or psychotherapists can modify degrees of focus, interest, relaxation, and engagement at the same time to enhance cognitive state.

5.2 Reinforcing positive cognitive states

According to the aforementioned observations, a person can use an ML-driven model to maintain a predicted level of Interest and Relaxation while achieving an optimal level of Stress. An ML model's insights can greatly aid Therapists in their efforts to comprehend and treat the psychosomatic disease. The connection between interest and relaxation may be used by a therapist to promote beneficial effects. The ML model produced by BCI can be applied in real-time and can shorten the time needed for therapists to treat patients for psychosomatic conditions. The validated model can be enhanced by the patient to improve their health and minimize expenditures associated with it.

The process of enhancing psychosomatic health can be accelerated and optimized using the ML model. In the process, value is created by the interaction of actors in healthcare, where this type of psychotherapy can be accomplished in a short amount of time with the use of the proposed experimental ML model. By scaling the model in the form of an App and Web portals, more people can get access to the healthcare ecosystem. Moreover, the well-being of an individual helps their respective organizations, enabling long-term growth. In line with self-tracking, people could reach a desired mental state (with or without help from therapists).

The approach mentioned in the given study would help people gain greater self-control and stay in the productive zone. This research offers the individual to increase their productivity and, in turn, enhance organizational performance. When combined with traditional statistical hypothesis testing, machine learning holds tremendous promise for the development of new models and can reveal interactions, hidden patterns of abnormal activity, brain anatomy and connections, and brain and physiological behavior systems as well as positive cognitive states.

6. Implications

6.1 Personalized approach

This study will help health practitioners analyze individual health indicators to customize their approach to enhancing psychosomatic health. EEG biofeedback can predict stress and energy level and can generate a signal that indicates a personalized level of engagement and focus of an individual. These signals would be generated by measuring the sleep patterns, stress levels, and circadian rhythms—that further helps individuals. With the help of a BCI device, the ML model would create nudges to forewarn these stress levels and additional mediators of well-being. When an individual would be able to measure the focus and engagement level, it would help him/her create work-life balance. This approach would give an individual an opportunity to rejuvenate their cognitive states of mind and the individual would be able to enhance their workplace productivity.

6.2 Enhanced self-efficacy

The technology in this study is wearable, and it can generate real-time data to improve individuals' well-being and offer personalized nudges. The ability conferred by the application of technology offers greater self-efficacy as the predictive power of ML will provide instant biofeedback. The data generated through ML could not only help individuals but health practitioners to provide "cognitive assistance" [75]. The noninvasive wearable accessories designed at a low cost will help the masses to personalize and reinforce positive cognitive states. Such machines will enhance individuals' self-efficacy and productivity; they will also reduce healthcare costs [76]. Healthcare services will be able to preserve the data generated through these devices and manage it by creating a healthcare ecosystem, and the data will offer portability. This entire process as a whole will reinforce positive cognitive states [52] for preventive healthcare.

6.3 Effective treatment

Brain-computer interface (BCI) will provide real-time data to give masses accessibility and portability to health-related data. Machine learning-driven models will reduce the time required for psychosomatic health treatments. Such models produced using A.I. will help individuals and therapists' access and re-evaluate the data at any time to reduce the cost and time. Thus, the machine learning model would expedite and optimize the process of augmenting cognitive states.

7. Limitations

As a data science-backed study it's not immune from the limitations on its own. Where the enrichment of results is dependent on the data quality and quantity. The accuracy of the data provided by BCI devices depends on the quality of the data captured by the subject. Hindrance in the data by the movement of the subjects during data collection or the unconscious reservations by the subject can provide garbage data to the ML model. Also, data modeling for this specific study utilizes features from the available dataset; hence its accuracy depends on certain boundaries of 5-channel brain-computer interaction [77]. By obtaining neural data from 14- or 32-channel EEG sensors, the same can be improved. Although the study maintained constant efforts to optimize data models, overfitting data in machine learning may lead to less clarity in the outcomes. Additionally, the application of data-driven analytical modeling in healthcare may have decreased diagnostic sensitivity. It may keep certain data that cannot be fitted into ML models out of focus. Such modeling may also appear complicated and multidimensional at the time, with a risk of disappearing and missing out due to observer variability.

In the future however application of ensemble modeling or neural networks, such study can be reinforced for greater reliability of results. Also, in the given study the constructs of well-being only focused on the "positive affect" of Hedonic well-being. While such a construct appears robust; it did not include other dimensions (such as happiness, hope, and self-acceptance) which may be due for consideration in future studies.

8. Conclusion

This book chapter extends the discussion on how digital technologies such as artificial intelligence (A.I.) and the Internet of medical things (IoMT) are changing health-related service provision and experiences. Their combination results in the effective sharing of health data and monitoring of real-time health, presenting personalized treatment options to the patient. The chapter reiterates the importance of technology—such as artificial intelligence as a component of healthcare services where a dynamic configuration of people, technologies, and positive cognitive states and highlights the link between mental and physical health. The study also reflects on how psychological health affects productivity at work. The research design makes extensive use of data science to fulfill its objectives that explore the role of positive emotions for the betterment of well-being using A.I. and reflect upon the co-created value in an organization through reinforced positive cognitive states brain-computer interfaces (BCIs) gather electroencephalography signals from the subjects and use machine learning to predict future cognitive states. The construct is pivoted on the significance of positive emotions, relating to stress, which has the potential to improve psychological well-being. The ML model predicts a person's stress levels as well as their link with "Interest" and "Relaxation." Continuous self-quantification fueled by positive emotions through "Self-tracking" and "Nudging" can improve psychological well-being. Moreover, the study offers significant insights into how positive cognitive states could enhance workplace productivity, ultimately resulting in greater organizational performance. We can infer that ML models can support psychotherapies to minimize time to therapy and increase patient access. In addition to reducing treatment time, reducing costs, and increasing patient access to the healthcare ecosystem, the outcome offers self-efficacy that can be effectively provided by the spatial flexibility and cognitive support generated from the iterative process. When dealing with AI-driven models, however, there are limitations including overfitting of data, diagnostic sensitivity, and observer variability.

9. Notes/thanks/other declarations

This book chapter reflects an experiment carried out during doctoral work and uses proprietary technology to draw presented insights.

Author details

Swapnil Morande[1*], Veena Tewari[2] and Kanwal Gul[1]

1 University of Naples, Napoli, Italy

2 University of Technology and Applied Sciences (Ibri), Oman

*Address all correspondence to: swapnil.morande@unina.it

References

[1] Kamran M, Bibi F, Rehman AU, Morris DW. Major depressive disorder: Existing hypotheses about pathophysiological mechanisms and new genetic findings. Genes (Basel). 2022;**13**(4):646. DOI: 10.3390/genes13040646

[2] Hidaka BH. Depression as a disease of modernity: Explanations for increasing prevalence. Journal of Affective Disorders. 2012;**140**(3):205-214. DOI: 10.1016/j.jad.2011.12.036

[3] Wang H, Tian X, Wang X, Wang Y. Evolution and emerging trends in depression research from 2004 to 2019: A literature visualization analysis. Frontiers in Psychiatry. 2021;**12**(October):1-20. DOI: 10.3389/fpsyt.2021.705749

[4] Søvold LE et al. Prioritizing the mental health and well-being of healthcare workers: An urgent global public health priority. Frontiers in Public Health. 2021;**9**(May):1-12. DOI: 10.3389/fpubh.2021.679397

[5] World Health Organization. Depression and Other Common Mental Disorders [Internet]. 2017. Available from: https://apps.who.int/iris/bitstream/handle/10665/254610/WHO-MSD-MER-2017.2-eng.pdf

[6] Schneiderman N, Ironson G, Siegel SD. Stress and health: Psychological, behavioral, and biological determinants. Annual Review of Clinical Psychology. 2005;**1**:607-628

[7] Haller H, Anheyer D, Cramer H, Dobos G. Complementary therapies for clinical depression: An overview of systematic reviews. BMJ Open. 2019;**9**(8):1-15. DOI: 10.1136/bmjopen-2018-028527

[8] Rojas G, Martínez V, Martínez P, Franco P, Jiménez-Molina Á. Improving mental health Care in Developing Countries through Digital Technologies: A mini narrative review of the Chilean case. Frontiers in Public Health. 2019;**7**(December):1-9. DOI: 10.3389/fpubh.2019.00391

[9] Wainberg ML et al. Challenges and opportunities in global mental health: A research-to-practice perspective. Current Psychiatry Reports. 2017;**19**(5):28. DOI: 10.1007/s11920-017-0780-z

[10] Jain FA, Walsh RN, Eisendrath SJ, Christensen S, Rael Cahn B. Critical analysis of the efficacy of meditation therapies for acute and subacute phase treatment of depressive disorders: A systematic review. Psychosomatics. 2015;**56**(2):140-152. DOI: 10.1016/j.psym.2014.10.007

[11] Slade M. Mental illness and well-being: The central importance of positive psychology and recovery approaches. BMC Health Services Research. 2010;**10**:26. DOI: 10.1186/1472-6963-10-26

[12] Payne A, Storbacka K, Frow P. Managing the co-creation of value. Journal of the Academy of Marketing Science. 2008;**36**(1):83-96

[13] Berry LL, Bendapudi N. Health care: A fertile field for service research. Journal of Service Research. 2007;**10**(2):111-122. DOI: 10.1177/1094670507306682

[14] Vargo SL, Lusch RF. From repeat patronage to value Co-creation in service ecosystems: A transcending conceptualization of relationship. Journal of Business Market Management.

2010;**4**(4):169-179. DOI: 10.1007/s12087-010-0046-0

[15] Secinaro S, Calandra D, Secinaro A, Muthurangu V, Biancone P. The role of artificial intelligence in healthcare: A structured literature review. BMC Medical Informatics and Decision Making. 2021;**21**(1):1-23. DOI: 10.1186/s12911-021-01488-9

[16] Saha S et al. Progress in brain computer Interface: Challenges and opportunities. Frontiers in Systems Neuroscience. 2021;**15**(February):1-20. DOI: 10.3389/fnsys.2021.578875

[17] Mariotti A. The effects of chronic stress on health: New insights into the molecular mechanisms of brain-body communication. Future Science OA. 2015;**1**(3):FSO23. DOI: 10.4155/fso.15.21

[18] Ahmed HU, Mari d JJ. The role of research in the prevention of mental disorders. Trends Psychiatry Psychother. 2014;**36**(1):1-2. DOI: 10.1590/2237-6089-2014-1000

[19] Ishihara-Paul L et al. Prospective association between emotional health and clinical evidence of Parkinson's disease. European Journal of Neurology. 2008;**15**(11):1148-1154

[20] Trudel-Fitzgerald C et al. Psychological well-being as part of the public health debate? Insight into dimensions, interventions, and policy. BMC Public Health. 2019;**19**(1):1-11. DOI: 10.1186/s12889-019-8029-x

[21] Boehm JK, Kubzansky LD. The heart's content: The association between positive psychological well-being and cardiovascular health. Psychological Bulletin. 2012;**138**(4):655-691. DOI: 10.1037/a0027448

[22] Malik M, Saidin N, Abd Wab R, Nordin N. Investigating the relationship between stress and psychological well-being among foundation students of UiTM. International Journal of Academic Research in Business and Social Sciences. 2020;**10**(14):93-101. DOI: 10.6007/ijarbss/v10-i14/7366

[23] Strizhitskaya O. Perceived stress and psychological well-being: The role of the emotional stability. Cognitive - Social, and Behavioural Sciences. 2019;**56**:155-162. DOI: 10.15405/epsbs.2019.02.02.18

[24] Yetton BD, Revord J, Margolis S, Lyubomirsky S, Seitz AR. Cognitive and physiological measures in well-being science: Limitations and lessons. Frontiers in Psychology. 2019;**10**(JULY):1-18. DOI: 10.3389/fpsyg.2019.01630

[25] Alexander R et al. The neuroscience of positive emotions and affect: Implications for cultivating happiness and wellbeing. Neuroscience and Biobehavioral Reviews. 2021;**121**:220-249. DOI: 10.1016/j.neubiorev.2020.12.002

[26] Park N, Peterson C, Szvarca D, Vander Molen RJ, Kim ES, Collon K. Positive psychology and physical health: Research and applications. American Journal of Lifestyle Medicine. 2016;**10**(3):200-206. DOI: 10.1177/1559827614550277

[27] Yang T, Gentile M, Shen CF, Cheng CM. Combining point-of-care diagnostics and internet of medical things (IOMT) to combat the Covid-19 pandemic. Diagnostics. 2020;**10**(4):4-6. DOI: 10.3390/diagnostics10040224

[28] Rejeb A, Treiblmaier H, Rejeb K, Zailani S. Blockchain research in healthcare: A bibliometric review and current research trends. Journal of Data, Information and Management. 2021;**3**(2):109-124. DOI: 10.1007/s42488-021-00046-2

[29] Shih JJ, Krusienski DJ, Wolpaw JR. Brain-computer interfaces in medicine. Mayo Clinic Proceedings. 2012;**87**(3):268-279. DOI: 10.1016/j.mayocp.2011.12.008

[30] Hazarika I. Artificial intelligence: Opportunities and implications for the health workforce. International Health. 2020;**12**(4):241-245. DOI: 10.1093/INTHEALTH/IHAA007

[31] Porter ME, Heppelmann JE. How smart, connected products are transforming competition. Harvard Business Review. 2014;**92**(11):64-88

[32] Thimbleby H. Technology and the future of healthcare. Journal of Public Health Research. 2013;**2**(28):e28

[33] Bughin J et al. "Tech for Good Smoothing Disruption, Improving Well- Being." McKinsey Global Institute. 2019;(May):1-78

[34] Čaić M, Holmlid S, Mahr D, Odekerken-Schröder G. Beneficiaries' view of actor networks: Service resonance for pluralistic actor networks. International Journal of Design. 2019;**13**(3):69-88

[35] McColl-Kennedy JR et al. The changing role of the health care customer: Review, synthesis and research agenda. Journal of Service Management. 2017;**28**(1):2-33. DOI: 10.1108/JOSM-01-2016-0018

[36] Graham S et al. Artificial intelligence for mental health and mental illnesses: An overview. Current Psychiatry Reports. 2019;**21**(11):116. DOI: 10.1007/s11920-019-1094-0

[37] Ahmed Z, Mohamed K, Zeeshan S, Dong XQ. Artificial intelligence with multi-functional machine learning platform development for better healthcare and precision medicine. Database. 2020;**2020**:1-35. DOI: 10.1093/database/baaa010

[38] Cannard C, Brandmeyer T, Wahbeh H, Delorme A. Self-health monitoring and wearable neurotechnologies. Handbook of Clinical Neurology. 2020;**168**:207-232. DOI: 10.1016/B978-0-444-63934-9.00016-0

[39] Hamet P. Artificial intelligence in medicine. Metabolism. 2017;**69**:S36-S40. DOI: 10.1016/J.METABOL.2017.01.011

[40] von Bertalanffy L. The meaning of general system theory. The quest for a general system theory. In: General System Theory. Foundations, Development, Applications. New York: George Braziller; 1968

[41] Capra F. THE WEB OF LIFE: A New Synthesis of Mind and Matter. USA: Anchor Books; 1996

[42] Jackson MC. Systems Thinking: Creative Holism for Managers. USA: John Wiley & Sons; 2016

[43] Bolton RN et al. Customer experience challenges: Bringing together digital, physical and social realms. Journal of Service Management. 2018;**29**(5):776-808

[44] Lupton D. The Quantified Self (Cambridge: Polity). USA: Wiley; 2016

[45] Ajana B. Digital health and the biopolitics of the quantified self. Digital Health. 2017;**3**:2-5. DOI: 10.1177/2055207616689509

[46] Yli-Kauhaluoma S, Pantzar M. Seeking connectivity to everyday health and wellness experiences: Specificities and consequences of connective gaps in self-tracking

data. Digital Health. 2018;**4**:2-8. DOI: 10.1177/2055207618779714

[47] Sharon T. Self-tracking for health and the quantified self: Re-articulating autonomy, solidarity, and authenticity in an age of personalized healthcare. Philosophy & Technology. 2017;**30**(1):93-121. DOI: 10.1007/s13347-016-0215-5

[48] Pantzar M, Ruckenstein M. The heart of everyday analytics: Emotional, material and practical extensions in self-tracking market. Consumption, Markets and Culture. 2015;**18**(1):92-109

[49] Ajana B. Personal metrics: Users' experiences and perceptions of self-tracking practices and data. Social Science Information. 2020;**59**(4):654-678. DOI: 10.1177/0539018420959522

[50] Chamorro-Koc M, Peake J, Meek A, Manimont G. Self-efficacy and trust in consumers' use of health-technologies devices for sports. Heliyon. 2021;**7**(8):e07794. DOI: 10.1016/j.heliyon.2021.e07794

[51] Sturts A, Gupta A. Wearable Fitness Tracking Improves Self-Efficacy for Exercise. Stratford: Rowan University; 2018

[52] Thaler RH, Sunstein CR. Nudge: Improving Decisions about Health, Wealth, and Happiness. India: Penguin; 2009

[53] Marchiori DR, Adriaanse MA, De Ridder DTD. Unresolved questions in nudging research: Putting the psychology back in nudging. Social and Personality Psychology Compass. 2017;**11**(1):1-13. DOI: 10.1111/spc3.12297

[54] Li M, Chapman GB. Nudge to health: Harnessing decision research to promote health behavior. Social and Personality Psychology Compass. 2013;**7**(3):187-198. DOI: 10.1111/spc3.12019

[55] Auf H, Dagman J, Renström S, Chaplin J. Gamification and nudging techniques for improving user engagement in mental health and well-being apps. Proceedings of the Design Society. 2021;**1**(AUGUST):1647-1656. DOI: 10.1017/pds.2021.426

[56] Feng S, Mäntymäki M, Dhir A, Salmela H. How self-tracking and the quantified self promote health and well-being: Systematic review. Journal of Medical Internet Research. 2021;**23**(9):e25171. DOI: 10.2196/25171

[57] Lorig KR, Sobel DS, Ritter PL, Laurent D, Hobbs M. Effect of a self-management program on patients with chronic disease. Effective Clinical Practice: ECP. 2001;**4**(6):256-262

[58] Anderson L et al. Transformative service research: An agenda for the future. Journal of Business Research. 2013;**66**(8):1203-1210

[59] Hirschle ALT, Gondim SMG. Stress and well-being at work: A literature review. Ciência & Saúde Coletiv. 2020;**25**(7):2721-2736. DOI: 10.1590/1413-81232020257.27902017

[60] World Health Organization. Promoting Mental Health: Concepts, Emerging Evidence, Practice. Geneva: WHO; 2004

[61] Ostrom AL, Parasuraman A, Bowen DE, Patrício L, Voss CA. Service research priorities in a rapidly changing context. Journal of Service Research. Apr 2015;**18**(2):127-159. DOI: 10.1177/1094670515576315

[62] Giuntella O, Hyde K, Saccardo S, Sadoff S. Lifestyle and mental health

disruptions during COVID-19. Proceedings of the National Academy of Sciences of the United States of America. 2021;**118**(9):e2016632118. DOI: 10.1073/pnas.2016632118

[63] Salari N et al. Prevalence of stress, anxiety, depression among the general population during the COVID-19 pandemic: A systematic review and meta-analysis. Globalization and Health. 2020;**16**(1):1-11

[64] Watson D, Clark LA. Measurement and mismeasurement of mood: Recurrent and emergent issues. Journal of Personality Assessment. 1997;**68**(2):267-296. DOI: 10.1207/s15327752jpa6802_4

[65] Cohen S, Gianaros PJ, Manuck SB. A stage model of stress and disease. Perspectives on Psychological Science. 2016;**11**(4):456-463

[66] Wersebe H, Lieb R, Meyer AH, Hofer P, Gloster AT. The link between stress, well-being, and psychological flexibility during an acceptance and commitment therapy self-help intervention. International Journal of Clinical and Health Psychology. 2018;**18**(1):60-68. DOI: 10.1016/j.ijchp.2017.09.002

[67] van Kraaij AWJ, Schiavone G, Lutin E, Claes S, van Hoof C. Relationship between chronic stress and heart rate over time modulated by gender in a cohort of office workers: Cross-sectional study using wearable technologies. Journal of Medical Internet Research. 2020;**22**(9):1-12. DOI: 10.2196/18253

[68] Satici B, Saricali M, Satici SA, Griffiths MD. Intolerance of uncertainty and mental wellbeing: Serial mediation by rumination and fear of COVID-19. International Journal of Mental Health and Addiction. 2020;**20**(5):1-12. DOI: 10.1007/s11469-020-00305-0

[69] Morse JM. Simultaneous and Sequential Qualitative Mixed Method Designs. USA: Qualitative Inquiry, SAGE Publishing; 2010. DOI: 10.1177/1077800410364741

[70] Mafuba K, Gates B. Sequential multiple methods as a contemporary method in learning disability nursing practice research. Journal of Intellectual Disabilities. 2012;**16**(4):287-296. DOI: 10.1177/1744629512462178

[71] Emotiv. The Introductory Guide to Neuroscience. 2021. Available from: https://www.emotiv.com/neuroscience-guide/. [Accessed: March 15, 2021]

[72] Faul F, Erdfelder E, Buchner A, Lang A-G. Statistical power analyses using G* power 3.1: Tests for correlation and regression analyses. Behavior Research Methods. 2009;**41**(4):1149-1160

[73] Morande S, Tewari V. Technology Management for Accelerated Recovery during COVID-19: A data-driven machine learning approach. Seisense Journal of Management. 2020;**3**(5):33-53. DOI: 10.33215/sjom.v3i5.445

[74] Segerstrom SC. Stress, energy, and immunity: An ecological view. Current Directions in Psychological Science. 2007;**16**(6):326-330. DOI: 10.1111/j.1467-8721.2007.00522.x

[75] Behera RK, Bala PK, Dhir A. The emerging role of cognitive computing in healthcare: A systematic literature review. International Journal of Medical Informatics. 2019;**129**(April):154-166. DOI: 10.1016/j.ijmedinf.2019.04.024

[76] Klassen RM, Klassen JRL. Self-efficacy beliefs of medical students:

A critical review. Perspectives on Medical Education. 2018;**7**(2):76-82. DOI: 10.1007/s40037-018-0411-3

[77] Rashid M et al. Current status, challenges, and possible solutions of EEG-based brain-computer Interface: A comprehensive review. Frontiers in Neurorobotics. 2020;**14**(June):1-35. DOI: 10.3389/fnbot.2020.00025